Foreword

By Nelson Stringer, M.D.

UTERINE FIBROIDS are the most common tumors of the female genital tract worldwide. When a woman is first diagnosed with fibroids, she is often faced with an unfamiliar diagnosis, with no independent roadmap to guide her decisions about treatment.

Unfortunately, many physicians in the United States do not offer women all the available options to treat fibroids. Even in the twenty-first century, physicians continue to debate the value of saving the uterus versus a hysterectomy . . . and as a result, too many women still have unnecessary hysterectomies for uterine fibroids. Any physician can perform a hysterectomy, but only a compassionate, concerned, and surgically skilled obstetrics/gynecology physician offers options other than a hysterectomy for the treatment of uterine fibroids.

But in terms of modern medicine, hysterectomy has never been the only option available to women with fibroids. The first successful removal of a fibroid without removing the uterus (myomectomy) occurred in 1845. As long ago as 1931, Dr. V. Bonney, a nationally respected obstetrics/gynecology physician who placed a high value on preserving the reproductive potential of women, wrote the following, "Since cure without deformity or loss of function must ever be surgery's highest ideal, the general proposition that myomectomy is a greater surgical achievement than hysterectomy is incontestable."

In more recent years, women's options have increased even further. Every woman, whether newly diagnosed with fibroids, or re-examining her options, must become knowledgeable about all the available treatment options for fibroids, and educated in the process of locating physicians that offer these options.

For instance, the development of new surgical instruments (operative hysteroscopes, laparoscopes, the ultrasonic scalpel, the Endo Stitch™ laparoscopic suturing device, powered laparoscopic morcellators, the On-Q™ Pain Management System), has radically expanded the conservative surgical treatment options for fibroids. I use these instruments to perform outpatient laparoscopic myomectomies on the majority of my patients who require surgical removal of their fibroids. In addition, new future oral medications for fibroids, such as Pirfenidone, will offer greater non-surgical treatment options. Women need a guide to navigate this often complex selection of options. I have attempted to achieve this process of educating women through my website, www.fibroid.com.

Ms. Skilling has also met the challenge of educating women in her new book, *The First Year™—Fibroids: An Essential Guide for the Newly Diagnosed*. This book offers a pragmatic, understanding, and logical guide for a woman to follow when she first discovers she has fibroids and will need treatment. The information in this book, including such topics as the benefits of diet and exercise, how to select a specialist, understanding insurance issues, exploring myomectomy, and uterine artery embolization, are invaluable to any woman with uterine fibroids.

The overall education and guidance provided in this book could make the difference between a woman obtaining a minimally invasive treatment option versus the standard hysterectomy offered by most physicians. If a woman follows the step by step approach presented by Ms. Skilling, when she contacts her physician, the process of resolving her problem with uterine fibroids will be less emotional, more informed, and most important, more surgically conservative. I highly recommend this book for any woman with uterine fibroids.

NELSON STRINGER, M.D., FACOG, is the director of the Fibroid Uterine Treatment Center and author of *Uterine Fibroids: What Every Woman Needs to Know*. He lives in Chicago, Illinois.

Introduction

FIBROIDS ARE the most common tumor of the human body. And yet they affect only women, growing as they do almost exclusively in the uterus. For this reason, the subject of fibroids is surprisingly intimate, sometimes embarrassing. A diagnosis is almost always shocking, if only because so few women know anything about fibroids before they're diagnosed themselves.

Fibroids are only recently getting to be a more mainstream topic of conversation, both among women and our health care providers. This is due in part to activism, in part to improving technology that has created more treatment options, and to the Internet, which has let large numbers of women find each other and share information about troubling symptoms, a fibroid diagnosis, and treatment recommendations.

You've picked up this book because you've received your own diagnosis of fibroids. It is not a life-threatening disease, but it can be a life-changing condition. If you have symptoms, they can affect every aspect of your life, from work, to travel, to the quality of your sexual experiences. Even if you don't have symptoms, confronting your decisions about treatment can open up questions about your goals, your female—and feminine—identity, your tolerance for uncertainty. There is a lot to think about.

There are a number of treatments for fibroids, ranging from lifestyle changes to invasive surgery, but as you'll see, your choice for treatment will be a highly individual, personal decision. How—or whether—you choose to treat your fibroids depends on your age, life goals, symptoms, and comfort level with each of the different treatment methods available.

One critical point that I want to state right up front is that having fibroids does not mean you have to lose your uterus. For many years, hysterectomy—the removal of your uterus and sometimes ovaries as well—was the treatment of choice for fibroids and their symptoms. But as we'll review in detail, there are many other choices you can make about treatment. In most cases, the decision to remove your uterus is yours and yours alone. A hysterectomy may prove to be appropriate, but it almost never needs to be the first choice treatment.

Your doctor can, and must, be a partner in your treatment decisions, but many aspects of having fibroids are completely in your control. This is because such seemingly unrelated choices as what you eat, how often you exercise, or how much stress you're feeling can affect your fibroids, the intensity of symptoms, and any anxiety or depression you feel about this new problem.

After you're more educated about your options, you may need to educate your health care providers about your treatment wishes, and if necessary, find a doctor who both understands your goals and has the skill to provide the treatment you prefer. By the time you've finished reading this book, I hope you'll realize that the only "bad" treatment decisions are those that are made without adequate information.

You have a lot to learn, and there is no reason for you to learn everything at once. It takes time before you can absorb it all. I know. I've had fibroids myself.

What happened to me

I had no pain, unusual bleeding, or problems of any kind when I scheduled my usual check-up in the summer of 1995. So it was with considerable surprise that I heard my gynecologist tell me that there was something wrong with my uterus. My doctor didn't diagnose me right away, but phoned the radiologist from her office and sent me, by cab, that minute, to get a sonogram. (If you haven't had a sonogram yet, you'll read a lot more about them on Day Two.) It was the radiologist, looking at the computer screen showing a picture of my pelvic cavity, who suddenly said, "Oh, my God! Look at these fibroids!"

I'm a fairly well-educated woman. I read the newspaper. I have informed friends. But I had never heard of these things, although they'd certainly gotten my radiologist all worked up. Later, back in my doctor's office, she talked to me about some of my immediate fears: cancer, surgery, infertility.

My doctor recommended that I have a myomectomy, a type of surgery that removes the fibroids and preserves the uterus. But I was scared. I was afraid that something would go wrong, and I would wind up getting a hysterectomy—that is, lose my entire uterus.

A few weeks before my myomectomy was scheduled, I canceled the surgery. And then I started finding out about fibroids.

I started by scheduling a second opinion with another doctor, and when that opinion was completely different, scheduling a third opinion, a fourth, even a fifth. Rather than clarify things, all this information made me more confused: Each doctor had a different idea of how to treat me.

And then I started talking to my friends and realized how many women I know have, or had, fibroids. It soon became clear how little information each of us had about this condition, and how reluctant most of us were to talk about it unless asked. So I began to do my own research. I began by reading, comparing reports from hundreds of sources. I talked with dozens of doctors and researchers who specialize in fibroid treatments and to women all over the country who had their own highly individual, personal stories of living with fibroids. In the meantime, I took the tactic I recommend as a first step for women who don't have symptoms, that is, "Watch and Wait." You'll read more about this in Week Three.

In 1998 I wrote my first book about fibroids, entitled *Fibroids: The Complete Guide*. In the year 2000, a few months after that book came out, and exactly five years after my initial diagnosis, my fibroids started growing so quickly that I had to seek more aggressive treatment. In the process, I got a fresh look at everything I needed to do to take care of myself physically, emotionally, and even financially. That's the experience—in addition to the newest information about fibroids and their treatments—that I will be sharing with you in this book.

How to use this book

I know that it can be overwhelming to learn about the many issues confronting you, and to think about your options, all at once. I've organized the information in this book by starting with the most essential things you should know right away, and then moving on to the more complex aspects of dealing with fibroids. Importantly, the treatment options are presented in priority order, from the gentlest natural alternatives to the most complete surgery.

Ideally, you would get this book the day you were diagnosed, but it may take days, weeks, or months before you find it or are ready to read it. Whenever you get the book—or open it—it's still okay to start with Day 1 and work your way through the chapters at your own pace.

Of course, if you like, you can choose to turn first to the pages describing the strongest treatments, just as you can choose to get surgery before trying other, less invasive, options. Simply put, my goal is to let you know that you do have options for treating your fibroids. In the end, the choice of what to do is yours, in partnership with a caring physician who understands and shares your goals. We'll talk about the importance of your own life goals in treating your fibroids in Week 3.

Each day or week or month in this book is divided into two sections, called Living and Learning. The Living sections of each chapter deal with the issues and problems of living with fibroids and their symptoms. Reading the Living sections, I hope you will feel that you're not alone; that the emotional reactions you'll probably go through are normal; and that while living with fibroids is sometimes hard, you have plenty of opportunities to take control, to improve both your symptoms, and your life.

The Learning sections of each chapter explain some of the more technical aspects of fibroids and their treatments, from the hormones that affect fibroids, to the medical techniques used to treat them. Some of the Learning sections, such as those in Days 1, 2, 3, and 4, will help you understand what fibroids are, how they grow inside your body, and how they affect you. Later Learning sections will give you the in-depth information you need to make an informed decision about each treatment option. If you prefer, start off by reading the Learning sections for the treatments that most appeal to you; later, you can go back and read other Learning sections to compare the pros and cons of all the other options available.

I will not prescribe

I am not a doctor, and I will not prescribe for you. For the most part, I've tried to keep my own preferences to myself, since I firmly believe that the course of treatment you decide on—whatever it is—is the best one for you, as long as you have done your research, consulted your heart, and are comfortable that you are making the best decision for your own life. No one else can make that decision for you, nor should they.

A word about genders: I have tried to use the prefixes "he" and "she" equally throughout the book when referring to doctors. The prefixes are intended to be interchangeable in all cases.

Where the focus is

This book is aimed at women going through their first year of living with fibroids. Most of you will not require invasive treatments in your first year. So although I discuss the pros and cons of various types of surgery, up to and including hysterectomy, this information is provided for your education and future reference. In the meantime, you can use the earlier sections in the book as an ongoing reference, to keep up to date on your lifestyle goals, and maintain records of your symptoms and treatments. There are many tools provided for your use throughout the book to monitor both your activities and the severity of the symptoms you have, if any, from your fibroids.

Keep on learning

Since you've decided to research your condition by picking up this book, I believe you're the type of person who wants to take an active role in your treatment. By the end of your first year with fibroids, I hope you will not only have a good grounding in current knowledge about fibroids and their treatments, but understand where you can go to continue the learning process, evaluate the announcements of news about fibroids and their treatments in the press, and share your learning with others.

At the end of Month 12, you'll see a selective list of books, magazines, newsletters, and organizations that I've found especially helpful for different aspects of living with fibroids. If you have access to the Internet, you'll also find a number of resources that can keep you updated on the latest news, treatments, and research, as well as places you can go to chat or trade information with other women.

New research information comes out regularly, on everything from genetic changes that may cause fibroids, to the devices and drugs that help treat them. Be cautious, though: There is a lot of hype and early enthusiasm for some developments, much of which is later tempered by experience. As knowledge about fibroids evolves, I hope what you learn from this book will enable you to keep up with the new advances, so you can work with your doctor to ensure that your own individual treatment plan evolves as well.

Nobody really knows how, or even why, fibroids develop, and none of the current treatments are perfect for everybody. The good news is that the more we talk, the more we learn, and the more we interact with our doctors and other health care providers, the better off we all will be. Remember, you've joined a community of women all over the world who understand what you're going through. You are not alone.

You're Diagnosed—
Now What?

YOU'VE BEEN to your doctor for a check-up. Perhaps it was time for your regular Pap smear, or perhaps you've had unusually bad cramps, abdominal pain, or abnormal bleeding. And during the examination, your doctor may have tightened her lips slightly, or raised her eyebrows, and told you that you have fibroids.

If you're like most women, you were immediately concerned: How severe is this diagnosis? What do I need to do next? Do I have cancer? Your doctor may have been able to answer all of your questions, some, or none of them. She may have told you that you have a number of options for treating, and dealing with your fibroids, or she may have simply told you that the "cure" is a **hysterectomy**.

In the first, confusing moments of hearing this new diagnosis, it can be hard to think of all the questions you should ask— or even to listen completely to what the doctor had to say. You need some time to absorb both the diagnosis and your doctor's recommendations . . . and to find out for yourself all about fibroids, how they can affect you, and what, exactly, you'd like to do about them.

By picking up this book, as well as taking advantage of other resources, you're taking the first, most crucial step for your care: you're taking the time to become informed about what fibroids are, what they are not, and what you can do to get the best treatment for yourself.

It's important to know that you're not alone: fibroids affect as many as 80 percent of women in America, as well as women all over the world. Fibroids are rarely a typical subject for conversation, but if you start mentioning them to your friends, you might be surprised how many people have a story to share with you.

Fibroids are a complex condition that affects individual women differently. Some women, like me, didn't know they had fibroids until they were in the doctor's office for a routine check-up. Many women experience heavy or abnormal bleeding. Other women experience pain, pressure, fatigue, gastrointestinal problems, or cramps. Women who are pregnant, or trying to become pregnant, may find that fibroids interfere with their ability to conceive, carry, or deliver via natural childbirth.

Your age and other individual circumstances can affect which treatment, if any, you choose to explore. For instance, if you still want to have children, your options will be limited to those that preserve possible future fertility. Conversely, if you're older, and in or near menopause, your changing hormones will affect how you'll approach certain treatments. Certainly, if you want to keep your uterus for any reason, you'll want to explore the options that allow you to do just that.

So who you are, and what your symptoms are, are a crucial part of what kind of treatment you will need, if any. Your doctor is a vital partner in your medical care, but may not have all the facts about fibroids at his or her fingertips, including the data on the newer treatment options. Most critically, your doctor won't know about your own health goals until you explain them. Your relationship with your doctor should be a respectful partnership—and it is up to you to help her or him out with the questions and information you both need to make a good decision on your behalf.

Your doctor should be able to tell you about your medical options (although as you'll see, there are non-medical treatment options as well), ranging from "Watch and Wait," to various types of surgery. Different symptoms can indicate different possible treatments, but be wary if your doctor provides only one option: hysterectomy. A hysterectomy, at a minimum, is the removal of your uterus. There are times when this surgery is appropriate, but for most women, it is not the first line of defense against fibroids. If you have just been diagnosed with fibroids and your doctor suggests that you have a hysterectomy, all you need to do is say, "I'll think about it." And then read the rest of this book.

On the first day you're diagnosed, you may feel overwhelmed, unnerved, ill-equipped to handle this new situation. You might panic; you might wonder what this thing is that has suddenly appeared in your body, in the most intimate part of your reproductive system, your uterus. It's normal to feel scared, uninformed, frustrated: A lot of women experience these kinds of emotions when they first hear the word "fibroids."

The first thing to do is take a long, deep breath. The first thing to know is that fibroids won't kill you. The second thing you need to do is decide to take care of yourself by finding out as much as you can about your fibroids, your options for treatment, and which of these options best suits your life and long term goals.

IN A SENTENCE:

> *Fibroids are a complex condition that affects individual women differently: Information will help you determine the best course of action for you.*

learning

Who Gets Fibroids?

JUST ABOUT any woman can get fibroids: Many standard sources say that 25 percent of women get them, and that's a big number all by itself. But at least one study shows that up to 80 percent of women may get fibroids, and about half of those women will have symptoms, like pain, pressure, or bleeding.

Scientists still don't know exactly why you might get fibroids. In a recent review of the scientific literature, The Agency for Healthcare Research and Quality reported that "Data were sparse on the natural history of fibroids." But we do know that you are more likely to get fibroids if your mother had them, or if you belong to certain ethnic groups. Researchers have found that many fibroids have a genetic abnormality, a trait that can be passed on from mother to daughter. Other studies have shown that women with a family history of fibroids, or a history of excessive bleeding, are much more likely to develop one or both of these problems than women with no family history.

If you're African-American, your chances of having fibroids are three times higher than women from other racial backgrounds (Caucasian, Asian, or Hispanic). African-American women also tend to develop fibroids at an earlier age, have larger and more numerous fibroids, and are more likely to have anemia and pelvic pain. Some doctors think that Jewish women may get fibroids at a higher rate than the "average," and there may be other groups of women who are more affected by fibroids than others.

Is there a certain age at which you can get fibroids? The short answer is no: I've spoken to women as young as nineteen as well as women well into their sixties, all affected by fibroids. But the late thirties and early forties seem to be the prime ages for women to be affected. A study of Japanese women, who generally have lower rates of fibroids than Western women, showed that the overall incidence of fibroids is about 10 percent; however, that rate doubles for women in their forties.

You can't control your age or the genes that you've inherited, but there are other possible risk factors that scientists have documented that you may be able to do something about. Weight could be one factor: A study done at the New England Deaconess Hospital showed that women who were at least 20 percent over their medically suggested weight were more likely to have fibroids. Another study showed that where you carry extra weight can also make a difference: women who had fat concentrated around the middle rather than thighs and hips had a significantly higher risk for fibroids.

But it's important to know that not every study confirms that heavier women are at greater risk for fibroids. And not all women with fibroids are heavy—far from it.

Other risk factors for fibroids include being sedentary or childless. On the other hand, for every study showing who's at risk for fibroids, there seems to be another study showing that those same types of people are not at risk. The greatest risk factor—one that none of us can avoid and few if any would want to—is our essential essence: We are female.

YOU CAN figure out if you have extra fat concentrated around your middle by taking a waist-to-hip ratio. Using a tape measure, measure your waist, and then your hips. Divide your waist measurement by your hip size: a 30-inch waist and 40-inch hips have a ratio of 0.75. Your risk increases if you have a 0.80 waist-to-hip ratio or higher.

What are fibroids?

Fibroids are firm, well-defined, round lumps of muscle, laced with blood vessels and surrounded by a tough, fibrous outer tissue. They tend to be light-colored—white, tan, or light pink. One doctor told me that fibroids resemble hard little rubber balls. The muscle that fibroids are made of is called "smooth muscle"; this is the type of muscle that forms your uterus.

The technical name for a fibroid is a **"monoclonal tumor."** The term "monoclonal" reflects the fact that each fibroid begins from a single cell: "mono" means "single" and "clonal" means, according to the Oxford American Dictionary, "an organism produced from one ancestor." Each fibroid was once a single cell in your uterus that somehow received the wrong message about how to grow and function.

Fibroids are also called **tumors, fibroid tumors, monoclonal tumors, fibromyomas, fibromas, myofibromas, myomas, leiomyomas, and leiomyomatas**. The fact that fibroids are called "tumors" does not mean that they are malignant; in fact, fewer than 1 percent of fibroids may ever become cancerous. A tumor is defined as an abnormal mass of tissue growing in the body: it may resemble normal tissue, but has no useful function, and in fact, grows at the expense of the body. But not all tumors are cancerous. In Month 7, we'll talk about the warning signs of cancer, and how doctors can track the changes that may signal danger. But for the moment, bear in mind that most fibroids are benign.

What makes fibroids grow?

How do fibroids go from being a single cell to a mass big enough for your doctor to feel in a routine exam? If anything, this is a bigger mystery than what causes fibroids in the first place, but there are several things that we do know:

Genetic Messages. Fibroids grow in the uterus, an organ whose cells are already genetically programmed to expand and multiply in pregnancy. Therefore, those cells already "know" how to grow; fibroids are probably uterine cells that have gotten the wrong message. Scientists have found several specific genes and chromosomes that can send the wrong growth message to uterine cells, and they are looking for more.

Estrogen. Studies have shown that women with fibroids have absolutely normal amounts of estrogen. But somehow, fibroid cells behave very differently than normal uterine tissue, using estrogen at a faster rate or attracting estrogen more than normal tissue. According to the Center for Uterine Fibroids, a division of Brigham & Women's Hospital in Boston, fibroids actually "have higher estrogen concentrations, bind more estrogen, have more estrogen receptors, and convert **estradiol** (a more active form of estrogen) to **estrone** (a less active form of estrogen) more slowly than normal **myometrium** (uterine cells)." This greater sensitivity of fibroids to estrogen may, in turn, have at least two other effects:

○ A gene called Wnt-7a controls the correct growth of uterine cells. Too much estrogen may make it impossible for this gene to function properly, allowing some uterine cells to expand to form fibroids.

○ Estrogen stimulates a hormone called **bFGF** (**basic fibroblast growth factor**): proper amounts of bFGF also control the growth of uterine cells. If this hormone is damaged, possibly as the result of a problem at the genetic level, it can make smooth muscle cells— the kind that make up fibroids—grow out of control.

Progesterone may also contribute to fibroid growth. The results of studies are contradictory: synthetic progesterone therapy has been shown to make fibroids smaller, larger, or have no effect at all. Anti-progesterones, however, such as the so-called "abortion pill," RU-486, have been shown to reduce fibroids.

Prostaglandins are a substance that the uterus produces, which, among other functions, promotes uterine contractions. Jane E. Brody, author of *The New York Times Book of Health,* suggests that prostaglandins may stimulate tumor growth.

Blood vessels. Fibroids feed on blood. Not only do your fibroids need blood to grow, but the same hormones that cause fibroid cells to grow may also make the blood vessels around them larger, creating an ever-greater supply of nourishment to the fibroids.

When fibroids die

When fibroids die, they're said to degenerate. This process is normal: Two-thirds of fibroids show some form of **degeneration**.

Fibroids degenerate when they outgrow their blood supply; they also usually degenerate after menopause, when reduced estrogen causes fibroids to shrink. When fibroids degenerate, they can **calcify**, meaning that they get harder, or liquefy; this is also called **necrosis**.

Degeneration can be a sign of infection; some doctors also think that it can signal malignancy, though there's disagreement as to whether the fibroid "turns into" cancer or a new, malignant tumor forms. Doctors who believe that degenerating fibroids can become cancerous think that it happens about 1 percent of the time.

There's no specific timing for degeneration, and you may notice no symptoms when it happens, or you might bleed more during your period, pass clots, get a low-grade fever, or feel a tenderness in your lower abdomen.

In some cases, degenerating fibroids cause severe pain. Physically, it's similar to a heart attack (both attacks are called **infarctions**): the fibroid is not getting enough blood to survive and a part of it dies. Unlike a heart attack, degenerating fibroids are not life threatening.

IN A SENTENCE:

> *Fibroids begin from a single cell in the uterus, grow, and sometimes die; they affect millions of women worldwide.*

living

Getting a Sonogram

IF YOUR doctor believes you have fibroids, the first test he or she is likely to recommend is a **sonogram**, or **ultrasound**. Sonograms are a relatively easy procedure; they may be a little uncomfortable, but they're generally painless and risk-free. The sonogram will literally provide a picture of your fibroids, showing how many you have, how big they are, and approximately where they are in your uterus.

Sonograms are usually performed by **radiologists**, often in a separate location from your doctor's office. You'll have to make an appointment: Your doctor or her staff might be able to do that for you.

When you have a sonogram, harmless, high-frequency sound waves are bounced against your pelvis to develop a picture of your uterus and any possible fibroids. You may be familiar with sonograms for another reason: They are the method of choice for checking up on a baby's progress in the course of pregnancy. In addition to fibroids, ultrasounds can detect the presence of polyps or other growths which can be missed during a regular physical exam.

There are two basic types of sonogram: a vaginal sonogram, which requires that the probe be inserted gently into your vagina, and an abdominal sonogram, in which the probe is run over the outer skin of your belly.

The American College of Preventive Medicine gives vaginal ultrasound the edge for providing a higher level of detail than abdominal ultrasound. However, some doctors feel that views taken from the inside don't show the top of your uterus adequately, and certain types of fibroids can be missed.

While sonograms cannot detect malignancy, regular sonograms can show whether your fibroids have grown since your last visit, and by how much. Every time you get a sonogram, ask for a copy of the report (the original will be sent to your doctor), as well as a copy of the sonogram pictures.

When you walk into your radiologist's office, you may have a feeling a little like stage fright. Like a novice performer, you're about to find out what you're made of. Just as in your doctor's examining room, you'll be on a padded table, feet propped up in stirrups. If you're having a vaginal sonogram, your radiologist will probably ask you to undress only from the waist down; you might find the appointment easier if you can avoid wearing a dress or pantyhose when you go, opting instead for an outfit that includes such items of clothing as trousers with knee-highs or socks.

The sonogram machine looks like a desktop computer. Instead of a mouse attached to a cord, there is a short, wand-like instrument, called the probe or **transducer**, that will send pictures of your pelvic cavity to the computer.

The radiologist will cover the probe with a latex covering (similar to a condom), lubricate it, and insert it into your vagina. Unless you're very dry inside, or very nervous, the insertion shouldn't hurt. Your radiologist may offer to let you insert the probe yourself, or if you like this idea, ask to do it. Once the probe is inserted, the radiologist will move it around inside you to get pictures of your uterus from various angles. Breathing deeply and slowly will help you relax your abdominal muscles, reduce irritation or pain from the probe, and make the procedure go more quickly.

The computer screen will show a series of images that the radiologist can explain. You can ask questions during the probe, or you may want to wait until all the data is collected. The great thing about a sonogram is that the results are immediate. While your radiologist is not the final arbiter of the results—that's your doctor's job—he or she can give you a report on the facts.

As the images appear, the radiologist saves them as pictures; these can be printed out and sent to your gynecologist. The computer will measure the fibroids, most often in centimeters. While this measurement can sound large, remember that two and a half centimeters equal one inch, about the length of your thumb from the knuckle to the tip.

When the radiologist or your doctor tells you the size of your fibroids, be prepared: Many doctors use the terminology of pregnancy to describe the size of fibroids. At eight weeks, for instance, a growing fetus is usually about one inch long: a one-inch fibroid then is sometimes called "an eight-week fibroid." This can be especially painful for women who are experiencing infertility, and many women, including me, prefer other common analogies for size, or simply pure measurements in inches or centimeters. Don't be afraid to ask your doctor to use descriptions which make you most comfortable.

What does the size of your fibroid signify? The answer in part depends on your symptoms. If you're bleeding heavily, even a very small fibroid can be a potential cause. Even without symptoms, fibroids as large as six inches can put pressure on the ligaments and muscles in your pelvis. (Here's a tip: If you decide to get sonograms on a regular basis, schedule the sonograms the same week of your cycle each time. Since fibroids may retain water, sonograms given the week before your period could show a larger uterus than during other times of the month . . . which could be mistaken for fibroid growth. It doesn't matter which week of your cycle you schedule sonograms, as long as you're consistent.)

If your radiologist decides that you need an abdominal sonogram, you'll need to fill your bladder before the sonogram, usually by drinking eight glasses of water—sixty-four ounces! Feeling "full" can take up to an hour. If you're like me, you may do a lot of squirming before you're allowed to empty your bladder again.

Except for this discomfort, the abdominal sonogram is simple: The radiologist slathers a cold blue lubricant over your distended belly and runs the probe over your skin. Everything else—the measurements, the pictures— are all the same as during a vaginal sonogram.

Drinking a lot of water in a short time can cool down your body temperature; you might feel really chilly afterwards. A hot cup of coffee or tea after the test is a simple but effective antidote.

Recent developments in sonogram technology include "Sonohysterography" (also called "Saline contrast sonohysterography," or "saline infusion sonohysterography (SIS)" or fluid sonography.) Sonohysterography involves filling your uterus with a small amount of saline solution to increase the contrast between your uterine lining and the cavity, allowing better visualization of any fibroids inside the cavity. You may experience cramping after this procedure. Discuss other potential risks, if any, with your doctor.

3-D imaging is another technique which provides an improved view of your uterus and fibroids. Instead of showing only the length and width of your fibroids, uterus, and ovaries, as sonograms do now, the new equipment measures volume, and offers a somewhat clearer image. Both of these procedures may be used to clarify results of a standard ultrasound.

IN A SENTENCE:

A standard sonogram is an easy, risk-free way to visualize your fibroids.

learning

What Your Uterus Looks Like, Where Your Fibroids Can Be

IN ORDER to understand your fibroids, it's helpful to know something about your uterus, the part of our bodies that Dr. Sherwin Nuland says has "mystified mankind for millennia." You may have seen diagrams that show the uterus seemingly suspended in space between your ovaries. It may not look like much in those black and white drawings, but in fact, it's an integral part of your pelvic anatomy.

Structurally, the uterus supports the other organs in your reproductive system, the vagina and ovaries. It also, by virtue of its place in your abdomen, helps support other internal organs, including your bladder and bowel, helping keep those organs firmly in their proper place.

The uterus is a rich source of hormones and other natural substances that may have wide-ranging effects on our bodies. In his book *The No-Hysterectomy Option*, Dr. Herbert Goldfarb writes that the uterus produces the natural painkillers called **beta endorphins**, that create "a mild euphoria and sense of well-being." Along with other parts of our reproductive systems, the uterus produces a unique and important natural antibiotic that in laboratory experiments killed even the infamous E. coli bacteria.

The uterus may also have a relationship to the health of your heart. Two of the substances the uterus produces are thought to help prevent heart disease, including **prostaglandins**, which cause smooth-muscle contractions, and **prostacyclins**, which cause blood vessels to relax.

The uterus also plays a little understood—and certainly little discussed—role in sex and orgasm. We'll talk about sex in detail in Month 3.

Despite the big role your uterus plays in your body, the size of an average uterus is fairly small. Two to four inches long, about two inches wide and one inch thick, it weighs only two to three ounces. If you've ever been pregnant, your uterus may be on the larger end of those dimensions. Of course, if you're pregnant now, or have fibroids, or other conditions such as **adenomyosis**, or **polyps**, it will be bigger still. (See Day 4 for a description of these other conditions.)

The uterus is a reddish-pink color, like the inside of your lips. It's shaped a bit like an empty balloon, with one open end, a narrow neck, and a rounded body that can expand easily.

The open end, with the rounded, protective collar, is the **cervix**. This is a small ring of muscle which forms the opening to the uterus and connects it with the vagina. The cervix is connected to the pelvic bones and ligaments, which help keep our pelvic organs in place.

Right after the cervix is the narrow neck of the balloon; this is the **isthmus**, a narrow passageway that connects the cervix and the wide part of the uterus.

This wide part is called the **fundus**; together, the fundus and the isthmus are called the body of the uterus, or the **corpus**. The body of the uterus is the part that grows during pregnancy; it's also the place you're most likely to find your fibroids. (In Latin, *fundus* means "farm," or "estate"—an interesting choice for the part of the body that nourishes children before they're born.)

At the rounded end of the fundus, the back of the balloon, two thin tubes come out from either side, like antennae. These are the **Fallopian tubes** (**oviducts**), that provide the pathway along which an egg travels from the ovaries to the uterus.

Most, though not all, fibroids form in the fundus, the large rounded part of the uterus. But there are still more distinctions in where fibroids are found. Remember, the inside of the uterus is hollow. But the surrounding

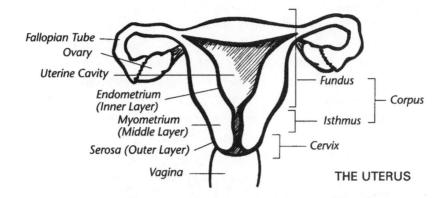

Fallopian Tube
Ovary
Uterine Cavity
Endometrium (Inner Layer)
Myometrium (Middle Layer)
Serosa (Outer Layer)
Vagina
Fundus
Corpus
Isthmus
Cervix

THE UTERUS

wall of the uterus is not a simple, single layer, like the pink plastic of a balloon. It is actually composed of three distinct layers, called the **serosa**, the **myometrium**, and the **endometrium**. Believe it or not, these terms will become very familiar as you learn more about how they relate to the names and locations of your fibroids.

Let's start with picturing the outside of the uterus. The thin, tough outer layer is the serosa. It protects the uterus and connects to the ligaments that support the uterus inside your pelvic cavity.

Fibroids on this outer layer can come in two shapes, either a ball on a stalk (**pedunculated**) or just a ball (**sessile**), embedded in the outer wall of your uterus. Because they form on the serosa, these fibroids are often

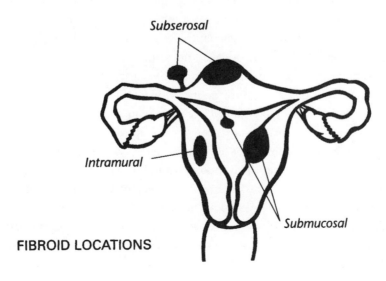

Subserosal
Intramural
Submucosal

FIBROID LOCATIONS

called **subserosal** fibroids. (Other names you may hear for these fibroids are **serosal**, **subserous**, or **subperitoneal**.)

Subserosal fibroids can push out the outer wall of the uterus, potentially pressing on other organs, such as the **ureters** or **bladder**. Sometimes they become big enough to push out against the wall of your abdomen, causing the kind of swelling that can make you feel, or even look, pregnant.

Pedunculated fibroids, growing on a stalk from the outer wall, can sometimes attach themselves to other organs or even the muscles in your pelvis. If these fibroids outgrow their original blood supply in the uterus, they may begin to draw blood from other organs, deserving their new name of **parasitic leiomyomata**.

Since subserosal fibroids aren't near the cavity, they generally don't affect your menstrual flow. As a rule, they don't even interfere with pregnancy. The main symptoms you can expect from these fibroids are pain, pressure, or gastrointestinal disturbances.

Under the serosa is the myometrium, usually called the uterine wall. This is a thick layer of smooth muscle, the same kind of muscle that your heart is made of. Like your heart, the uterine wall contracts and expands according to signals sent by your body. You feel these contractions most often during your period, during childbirth, and during sex.

Fibroids in the uterine muscle are called **intramural** or **interstitial** fibroids (*intra* means "within"; *mural* refers to the wall). These are the most common fibroids. As intramural fibroids expand, they make the uterus feel larger; depending on how deep in the muscle they are, they can distort the cavity of the uterus or press out against the outer wall toward the pelvis.

Small intramural fibroids may cause no symptoms at all. But as they grow, or as more fibroids form, they can make the cavity of the uterus larger, resulting in heavier bleeding during your period.

If intramural fibroids grow quite large, they can start pressing on the other organs in your pelvis, or cause heavier cramps during your period.

Under the myometrium is the endometrium (also called the uterine **mucosa** or the uterine lining). The endometrium is the layer that surrounds the cavity of the uterus; it's also one of the areas most likely to be noticeably disrupted by fibroids. The endometrium itself has two layers: The first is a thin layer which grows new blood vessels every month; second is the endometrial lining, the layer of blood that builds up every month in preparation for pregnancy, or is shed when we have our periods.

Fibroids that grow from the uterine lining are called **submucous**. Although they're the least common (5 percent of fibroids), they produce some of the most obvious symptoms. Since they interfere with the blood vessels in the lining, even a tiny submucous fibroid can cause heavy bleeding and prolonged periods. These fibroids are also the ones that can interfere with pregnancy the most.

Like fibroids that grow on the outer layer of the uterus, fibroids that grow in the lining come in two forms, either nestled into the lining like a ball (sessile) or growing from a stalk (pedunculated). The stalk of a pedunculated fibroid is rooted in the lining, while the fibroid itself hangs into the cavity like a lightbulb dangling from the ceiling. Since pedunculated fibroids actually take up space inside your uterus, these are also called **intracavity fibroids**.

> **A RARE** fourth type of fibroid is found on the cervix; this is known as a **cervical myoma**. If you go for regular check-ups to your ob-gyn, these growths should be found in the most basic beginning stage, as **dysplasia**, or abnormal cell formations, and removed before they grow. Often your doctor can remove these cells during an office visit, although the procedure can be momentarily painful.

Knowing where your fibroids are growing is important, because where they are can make a difference as to how they affect you and what treatments you may be able to have. For instance, fibroids in the cavity of your uterus are easier to reach surgically than fibroids in the wall. Of course, as fibroids grow, they may encroach on more than one part of the uterus.

Also, don't be surprised if you have more than one fibroid. The average woman with fibroids has five or six, growing either in clusters or singly. Each fibroid grows at its own pace though, so it's possible you could have one large fibroid along with several smaller ones, or even microscopic ones.

IN A SENTENCE:

> *The uterus is a complex organ; where your fibroids develop can affect both your symptoms and your treatment options.*

DAY **3**

living

Take Inventory of Your Lifestyle

THERE ARE many reasons that fibroids occur naturally—as a result of your genes or changes in how your hormones interact—but did you know that fibroids can thrive in certain environments? It's true . . . and you have a certain amount of control over that environment through what you eat and drink, how active you are, even how much sleep you get.

We'll discuss specific plans for diet and exercise later this week, in Day 5, where we'll learn about foods that help and foods that can hurt, and Day 7, where we'll talk about how exercise can help you manage the effects of your fibroids.

But the first step in learning how you can take charge of your daily habits is to take a very realistic look at what you do now, in as much detail as you can manage.

Like you, I expect, I have long tried to modify my lifestyle through healthier eating and trying to incorporate more exercise into my weekly routine. I was frustrated that I wasn't losing weight, despite what I thought of as a healthy lifestyle. So I tried going on the Weight Watchers™ program, and took their advice on keeping track of everything I ate. Keeping a daily food diary quickly showed me the difference between my perception and reality: suddenly, one day of my sort-of healthy diet looked like two days worth of calories! Now I had the information I needed to start making choices that would make a difference.

This same type of daily record-keeping can help you determine whether your lifestyle is going to help or hurt your fibroids. The point of this step is *not* to edit or change anything you're doing, at least not at first. What you want to do is give yourself the most realistic perspective on your daily life.

This is a good day to create your personal "Lifestyle and Symptoms Indicator." This will include the symptoms you experience, if any, as well as what you eat, medicines you take, how often you exercise, and what might have stressed you out. If you decide to do this, don't judge what you did; just write it down. Over time, you may notice that certain things you do in your daily life affect your symptoms, positively or negatively. If you do see a pattern, you can experiment with making changes that will accentuate the positive. Since nobody has to see your daily record but you, you can afford to be honest. And honesty is important, even if it's painful, embarrassing, or just plain irritating. Remember, the truth can set you free—if you let it.

On the next page is one way you might want to set up your Lifestyle and Symptoms Indicator. It's important to write down everything consistently, so you can develop a realistic picture, for instance, of how often you *really* work out, or how much stress you've got in your day.

Your Lifestyle and Symptoms Indicator can be as simple as noting any problems you feel on your calendar. If you have access to a computer, you might want to type in all the categories and then print out pages that you can put in a notebook and fill in by hand every day. Or you can fill in your daily entries on your computer, printing out the finished pages to re-read later. Certainly, old-fashioned handwriting on a legal pad or spiral-bound notebook will also work perfectly well.

Once you get in the habit, it won't take long to fill this out. Try setting aside ten minutes before bed, right after you brush your teeth, to make sure you fill out all the information that's important for that day.

IN A SENTENCE:

> *Keeping track of your lifestyle will help you target areas for healthy changes.*

MY FIBROIDS LIFESTYLE
AND SYMPTOMS INDICATOR

Day: *Monday*

Date: *January 1*

Symptoms (if any), and intensity (mild/moderate/severe)

Bleeding

Cramps

Pressure

Other

What I ate today: *Breakfast, lunch, dinner, snacks*

What I drank today: *Especially coffee, sodas, juice, alcoholic drinks*

What stressed me out: *At work, home, elsewhere*

Medicines I took/prescription: *Examples: birth control pills, thyroid medication*

Medicines I took/non-prescription: *Examples: aspirin, cold or allergy remedies*

Vitamins I took: *Example: Multivitamin*

Herbs I took: *Example: Ginkgo biloba*

Exercise I did: *Example: treadmill*

How long I worked out: *Example: 20 minutes*

How much sleep I got last night: *Example: 6 hours*

What Are the Symptoms of Fibroids?

NOT EVERY woman with fibroids has symptoms. But if you do, it can be a scary experience. Severe symptoms can limit your activities both at work and at home: in the United States alone, fibroids are thought to be responsible for 5–10 million lost workdays each year.

The most common symptoms are abnormal uterine bleeding, pain, or pressure in your lower abdomen. But depending on where your fibroids are, they can cause a wide range of additional problems, including heavy bleeding or bad cramps during your period, loss of your period, anemia, pain during sexual intercourse, pain in your lower back, difficulty urinating or increased need to urinate, constipation, or fatigue. If you're pregnant, or trying to get pregnant, fibroids can sometimes cause infertility, miscarriage, or preterm labor.

It's important to know that these symptoms are not limited to fibroids; some of them could be the signal for other problems, such as **endometriosis**, **polyps**, or **adenomyosis**—and equally important to know that doctors could mistake one of these common conditions for fibroids. We'll review these other conditions on Day 4.

Let's look at the details of the major symptoms of having fibroids.

Uterine bleeding

Heavy bleeding is one of the most common symptoms, affecting about a third of all women with fibroids. Many women with fibroids experience extra heavy periods, but any type of abnormal bleeding is possible. In fact, uterine bleeding is one of the most common gynecologic problems doctors see: It accounts for approximately 15 percent of office visits and 25 percent of gynecologic operations.

There are a number of terms used to describe different levels of bleeding. Even though some of the terms may sound daunting, notice that some describe perfectly normal menstrual periods. Of the terms listed below, only three—menorrhagia, hypermenorrhea, and metromenorrhagia—refer to excessive bleeding.

- **Ovulatory bleeding**: Your normal period, occurring every 21–40 days.
- **Intermenstrual bleeding** (breakthrough bleeding): Bleeding between your periods.
- **Menorrhagia**: Prolonged, heavy flow during your period.
- **Hypomenorrhea**: Light periods at normal intervals.
- **Hypermenorrhea**: Heavy periods at normal intervals.
- **Polymenorrhea**: Periods at shorter than usual intervals, every twenty-one days or less.
- **Oligomenorrhea**: Long gaps between your periods, from forty-one days to six months.
- **Amenorrhea**: You've had no periods for at least six months.
- **Metromenorrhagia** (or metrorrhagia): Heavy bleeding at unpredictable intervals
- **Spotting**: Light, irregular flow, including light pink or brown staining.
- **Postmenopausal bleeding**: Bleeding occurring more than one year after menopause

On average, a menstrual cycle lasts twenty-eight days, including four days of bleeding. The average blood loss is about 1.2 ounces, or roughly the amount of liquid held by two tablespoons. Heavy bleeding is a relative term. While someone who often has a light period may notice heavier flows, it may not be dangerous. One way to tell if you're bleeding heavily is to keep track of the duration and flow of your period: bleeding for more than seven days or using more than ten pads or tampons per day during the menstrual cycle is considered excessive. Some variation in your period is normal, but if you have been bleeding heavily for three months or more it is definitely time to see a doctor.

While heavy bleeding is unpleasant, messy, and often a source of worry, it is not considered dangerous unless it's heavy enough to cause **anemia**. The amount of blood loss in a single day that could start causing anemia is between two and three ounces, or about a quarter of a cup. Anemia can be diagnosed very easily after a simple blood test.

If you are bleeding heavily, it's often because your fibroids have interrupted the normal way your body works. Fibroids seem to cause excess bleeding in several ways:

○ Fibroids in the wall or lining of your uterus can interrupt its normal, rhythmic contractions, meaning it can't squeeze shut the blood vessels in the lining as well as usual.
○ The blood vessels that feed fibroids may become so large that the normal clotting action of the blood is no longer effective.
○ A protein that reduces muscle tone may relax the fibroid muscle, allowing blood vessels to bleed more freely.

Not every fibroid causes heavy bleeding; intramural fibroids, for instance, generally don't cause heavy bleeding because of their position away from the cavity of the uterus. The worst culprits for bleeding are generally the submucous, those fibroids located in the lining of your uterus.

But before you or your doctor automatically assume that your fibroids are causing your bleeding problem—or that they're the only reason—be sure that you can rule out any other causes. Doctors have identified over thirty possible reasons for abnormal bleeding. In addition to fibroids, these include endometriosis, adenomyosis, and **polycystic ovaries**. **Ectopic pregnancy** can cause bleeding, as can complications from abortions or sexual trauma, such as rape; sometimes contraceptives can cause the problem, including birth control pills or IUDs. Other things to have checked out are the possibility of any infections, such as **candida**, and blood clotting problems (see von **Willebrand's Disease**, on Day 4). Many women also experience something doctors call "dysfunctional" bleeding, that is, bleeding without an obvious physical cause.

If you're in the age range that is now known as the **perimenopausal** years—about five to ten years before full menopause sets in—bleeding could also be due to the hormonal changes common during this time. This is in addition to the possible causes listed above.

Heavy bleeding may also be caused by problems that seemingly have nothing to do with your reproductive system, including liver or thyroid ailments, even leukemia or other cancers. It could be a sign of endometrial or cervical cancer, especially after menopause. While fibroids are not usually malignant, bleeding in some women (not all) can be a symptom of cancer. You can go to a **gynecological oncologist** (cancer specialist) to rule out any malignancies. Although the majority of abnormal bleeding comes from the uterus, you'll need a good physical examination to rule out vulvar, vaginal, and cervical or other problems.

If you have already experienced menopause, any bleeding is a good reason to go see your doctor. If you're taking **Hormone Replacement Therapy (HRT)** of any kind, you should be especially careful to note when the bleeding occurs in order to see if the bleeding approximates a menstrual cycle. As we grow older, the possibility of reproductive cancer becomes higher: 10 percent of women with postmenopausal bleeding have cancer, and this percentage increases with age. The more common causes of bleeding in this age group—and the explanation for up to 90 percent of postmenopausal bleeding—are benign conditions, such as vaginal or endometrial atrophy.

Cramps

Cramps are more than just an inconvenience. As many as one in ten women are temporarily disabled during their periods. And while we may think of menstrual pain as being routine, there is evidence that pain may weaken the immune system, lowering your resistance to all kinds of disease.

There are two kinds of cramps, also known as **dysmenorrhea**.

○ Primary dysmenorrhea is caused by prostaglandins, the hormones which make your uterus contract during menstruation. If the contractions are very strong, they can temporarily cut off the blood supply to your uterus. This deprives your uterus of oxygen, which in turn creates the pain you feel. It's possible that women who have truly painful cramps produce higher than normal amounts of prostaglandins. Most women who have primary dysmenorrhea have had it most of their adult lives.

○ Secondary dysmenorrhea describes cramps that may have started later in life and gotten worse over time. These cramps can usually be traced to an obvious cause, such as fibroids, pelvic inflammatory disease (PID), or endometriosis. These cramps aren't limited to your monthly period; they also occur during intercourse, or even during times of the month when you're not menstruating.

Use your Lifestyle and Symptoms Indicator to track when and how often your cramps occur. This can help you and your doctor pinpoint more accurate treatment methods.

Pain or pressure

The uterus is supported by a network of ligaments and muscles. As the fibroid grows and the uterus stretches, more strain is put on the muscular support structure that you have in your abdomen. It's similar to adding more and more weight to a hammock. The more weight you add, the more the

Anemia

IF YOU'RE bleeding too much, you're a candidate for anemia. When you lose blood, you lose iron, and without iron, your body doesn't use oxygen as efficiently. That can lead to a consistent feeling of low energy: you might feel slower than usual, easily tired, or listless.

And it's not just heavy periods that can make you anemic. Fibroids seem to need more blood than normal tissue, and studies show that arteries actually grow to feed the fibroids more—taking vital nutrients away from the rest of your body.

fabric is pulled; that's what can happen to your pelvic muscles when they have to support a heavy fibroid. At worst, fibroids can cause **uterine prolapse**, the term for when your uterus is forced down and into your vagina.

Pressure from a large uterus can also affect other pelvic organs. An enlarged uterus can squeeze the ureters, the tubes that transport urine from the kidneys. This can reduce flow, and in serious cases—if urine backs up into the kidneys—can lead to kidney infection and damage. In extreme cases, large fibroids can result in kidney failure. The symptoms you might feel include increased need to urinate, sometimes badly, sometimes without being able to go at all. On the other hand, you might experience **urinary incontinence**, the inability to hold back your urine, when you sneeze or laugh or exercise hard.

A larger uterus can also put pressure on your bowel, which may mean that your body can't eliminate waste properly. This can create such symptoms as irritability, an uncomfortable feeling of fullness in your abdomen, constipation, and in extreme cases, intestinal obstruction.

Large fibroids can also put pressure on the nerves or blood vessels. Compressed blood vessels can lead to such problems as varicose veins, swelling in your legs, and hemorrhoids; pressure on pelvic nerves can cause painful feelings in the lower back, one or both legs (sciatica), or numbness in the legs.

Fatigue

Fibroids can make you tired. In one study, 70 percent of women with fibroids experienced fatigue. First, as we discussed, fibroids demand a constant supply of blood to stay alive; they're little thieves, stealing parts of your blood supply that your body had other plans for. If your fibroids are causing you to bleed heavily, you may also be losing too much blood and iron, which can also create fatigue.

The second reason fibroids can be fatiguing is that they're an extra weight. Not when they're small, but if they get to the size of a four-month pregnancy, for instance, you're carrying around a couple of extra pounds just in fibroid weight. Some women claim that fibroids caused them to put on even more weight, and while that's not documented scientifically, it's an article of faith for the women who go through it. Even if it's not much, even if fibroids only add an extra five pounds—your body has to work harder.

Third, if you're spending time worrying about having fibroids or treating them, that too can be tiring. Anxiety uses energy.

Difficulty during sex

For some women, fibroids can make sex—or even the prospect of sex—less pleasant, even impossible. Fibroids can cause a variety of problems, including pressure, pain during penetration, a feeling that the uterus is shifting around, and uterine, ovarian, or back pain. During intercourse your fibroids can press up against adjacent organs like the bladder or **rectum**. They won't cause any damage, but the feeling may be distracting. Fibroids can also affect your ability to have an orgasm by preventing the uterus from being able to elevate, expand, or create contractions.

Fibroids can also make the choice of birth control a significant problem. Since birth control pills may cause fibroids to grow, they may not be an option. If your fibroids have distorted the shape of your uterus, by tipping it back or changing the shape of the cervix, a diaphragm isn't an option either, since it can't be fit properly and can also cause pain or pressure.

Having fibroids may mean you'll choose not to have sex at all, because of bleeding, pain, fatigue, or plain old lack of desire brought about by any, or all, of the above. Of course, anything that affects your sex life can affect your self-esteem, feelings of femininity, and your relationship, if you're in one. Worst, you can start feeling like there's something wrong with you as a person.

You'll see more about fibroids and sex in Month 3.

Infertility and miscarriage

Fibroids can create an inhospitable atmosphere in a woman's uterus, making it difficult to conceive. If you do become pregnant, fibroids can pose different problems. Fibroids in the cavity are known culprits in miscarriages, as well as premature labor and other complications.

In studies of women who have fibroids, there's a high rate of infertility and spontaneous abortion. In her book, *Having Your Baby: A Guide for*

African-American Women, Dr. Hilda Hutcherson says that "the presence of fibroids can make it very difficult or even impossible to get pregnant."

While fibroids can affect women of any age, they are most often an issue for women in their thirties and forties. And pregnancies in women over thirty-five quadrupled in the decade between 1980 and 1990. These "older" women—older than thirty-five—are the fastest-growing group of women seeking treatment for infertility.

We'll talk about pregnancy in more detail in Month 5.

IN A SENTENCE:

Fibroids can cause one, many, or no symptoms at all.

How to Talk About Having Fibroids

IT'S DAY 4 after your diagnosis. Your natural instinct may already have been to confide in someone: your spouse or significant other, your mother, your best friend. And maybe you got the kind of support you wanted and needed. But many women don't get that reaction from the first person they talk to, and they stop talking. Or it may be that you haven't found the words, or the person, to talk with yet—and you're living with your fears and feelings alone.

Let's choose today to break out of that box, if need be.

Fibroids are funny things to talk about. First of all, a lot of us are reluctant to talk about our gynecological problems. We all have our own comfort levels regarding what we'll reveal about ourselves, and to whom, and fibroids may seem too intimate, too personal to discuss.

And then there's the mystery factor. If your friends or family don't understand what fibroids are, they may not know how to comfort you or provide the support you need.

So today you have two jobs: first, to nominate your personal Fibroid Support Team, and second, to learn how to make sure you get the support you want, need, and deserve.

Let's start with the first assignment, that is, deciding who you would like to be on your team. Start by filling out this list so that you can visualize who is in your life and who you can depend on for intelligent, caring support for your fibroid treatment. Write in as many names as you would like to in each of the appropriate categories (you can skip the categories that don't apply to you).

Spouse or partner: _____

Parent(s): _____

Other family members: _____

Long-term friends: _____

Friends you see or talk to every day: _____

Friends you see less often but are fond of: _____

Friends at work or school: _____

Friends at your church, synagogue, mosque, or temple: _____

Friends from community groups: _____

Neighbors: _____

When you've finished writing your list, it might look something like a list of people you'd invite to a big party. And if you're like me, you ask people to bring things to the parties you throw . . . somebody can be counted on to make an ambitious dessert, while someone else can stop and pick up ice at the corner deli, but they all contribute to the party's success.

So think about your assignment list, and what you'd like each of the people you nominated for your Fibroid Support Team to do. You can choose more than one person for each assignment. Start with the list below, and add things that apply just to you:

ASSIGNMENT	NOMINEE
Heart-to-heart talk about what you're going through	_____
Company for your next visit(s) to the doctor	_____
Go with you tomorrow (Day 5) to the market	_____
Go with you the next day (Day 6) to the drugstore	_____
Make an exercise date	_____
Ask if they know anything about fibroids	_____
Ask for ob/gyn recommendation	_____

Ask for help doing Internet research	_____
Give you a hug	_____
Go out for dinner	_____
and . . . _____	_____
_____	_____
_____	_____

Each of these assignments is valuable, but most important is making sure you have at least one person to confide in; this may not be the person you'd most expect, such as your partner or your mother. But even if the first person you talk to disappoints you in some way, don't give up. Somebody is out there who will listen to you and let you talk about your feelings.

You also may need to help your nominee before she can help you: Not everyone reacts the same way, or just the way you might hope. Let your friends and loved ones know what you need. Most of them will do their best to give you what they can. (For those who don't live up to your expectations, try not to be angry; that's why you have a number of names on your Support Team.)

If you need more incentives to take this step, look at these facts:

○ Talking out your thoughts is good for you. Studies show that feelings of stress and isolation actually depress your immune system.
○ A study of breast cancer patients showed that the women who were most able to share their feelings with others had a significantly higher level of well-being.
○ Caring conversation can change the physical circuitry of your brain, literally creating connections for more positive thoughts and feelings.

In addition to the family and friends that you've nominated to be on your Fibroid Support Team, there are some other resources you can draw on. The first is *therapy*. Therapists can sometimes help you sort out issues that ob/gyns and your circle of friends cannot: fears about more serious illness, fear of certain treatments, questions or concerns about your sexuality and relationships. You may benefit from a few visits; you may find caring support in a longer-term relationship with a trained social worker, psychologist, or psychiatrist.

A *house of worship* can also provide caring community. Many congregations have a weekly prayer list; the names of people needing prayers for healing are read out loud during services. There may be weekly healing services that take place outside of regular hours of worship. If your congregation doesn't currently offer this, and it sounds like something you would like, consider asking, or forming one yourself. There will be other people who would appreciate it, too.

Last, there's that great resource, *the Internet*. There are several resources out there for women with fibroids, and by the time you read this, there may well be more. You can even start your own group, and you don't have to be a computer genius to do it. (You'll find a number of resources, including many on the Internet, listed in Month 12.)

One caution: It's great to listen and be open to what other women have to say, but consider whether their situation is the same as yours. The Internet is an incredible source of information, but it can also attract people who need to discuss their problems. Their issues and yours may not be the same . . . and you may get a distorted sense of whether a treatment works, since success stories don't always find their way into the electronic world.

IN A SENTENCE:

> *Choosing a Fibroid Support Team can make sure you get the caring you want, need, and deserve.*

learning

When It Isn't Just a Fibroid

AS WE saw yesterday, in Day 3, there are several conditions that may cause the same types of symptoms as fibroids. It's important for you and your doctor to be able to rule out these other causes before proceeding with treatment, especially if that treatment includes surgery. On the other hand, if fibroids don't seem to be the reason for your symptoms, you shouldn't assume that your problems have no physical cause.

The conditions that can mimic—or co-exist with—fibroids include polyps, endometriosis, adenomyosis, and a blood disorder known as von Willebrand's disease.

Polyps

Polyps are fleshy growths that grow from the lining of the uterus into the uterine cavity. (In this, they are like pedunculated submucosal fibroids; see Day 2.) Polyps are almost always benign. According to the Center for Uterine Fibroids, malignancy has been reported in only six out of every thousand cases (0.6%).

Polyps are almost as common as fibroids; what's more, they cause fully 25 percent of the cases of abnormal bleeding. Polyps can affect you at any stage of life: they can cause prolonged, heavy bleeding before menopause, bleeding after menopause, and breakthrough bleeding in women on hormone therapy. So even though you have fibroids, if you're bleeding, you should find out if you have polyps as well.

Since polyps are almost always in the uterine lining, they're relatively easy for a doctor to remove through a type of outpatient surgery called **hysteroscopy** (see Month 6).

Endometriosis

This is another common disorder, affecting about nine million women. Endometriosis is second only to uterine fibroids as the most frequent cause of surgery in premenopausal women, accounting for 18 percent of hysterectomies every year.

If you have endometriosis, pieces of your uterine lining have somehow migrated to other parts of your pelvis. The symptoms of endometriosis include pain, difficulty during sex, irregular bleeding, and infertility. After ruling out other conditions, such as fibroids, the only definitive test for endometriosis is **laparoscopy**, which allows the doctor both to see whether there's a problem and then to take a **biopsy** in order to examine the tissue for evidence of disease. We'll discuss more about laparoscopy and biopsies in detail in Month 6.

Adenomyosis

Adenomyosis is a condition similar to endometriosis, in which parts of the endometrium (the uterine lining) somehow migrate away from where they belong. In adenomyosis, the lining is somehow pushed deeper into the uterine wall. Although adenomyosis is not thought to be cancerous, it can cause a lot of pain and abnormal bleeding.

Like fibroids and endometriosis, the origins of adenomyosis are somewhat mysterious. That is, nobody knows how or why you might get it. It's also an amazingly common condition; about 20 percent of women have symptoms, and microscopic analysis of uterine specimens reveal that as many as 65 percent of women have it. As a rule, adenomyosis tends to show up in women between forty and fifty years old, mostly in women who have had at least one child.

Adenomyosis often appears in conjunction with other problems; 50 percent of the women with adenomyosis also have fibroids; many have endometriosis or polyps. As a result, diagnosing and treating adenomyosis can be complicated. Like endometriosis, the only certain way to get a diagnosis of adenomyosis is through a surgical biopsy.

von Willebrand's Disease

Von Willebrand's disease, like **hemophilia**, is an inherited bleeding disorder which makes your blood clot more slowly than normal: it affects about three out of every hundred women (3 percent). However, if you have very heavy periods, the possibility of your having von Willebrand's increases up to 15 percent. There's a small possibility of other clotting problems being present, including factor XI deficiency, platelet dysfunction, or presence of the gene for hemophilia.

If you have von Willebrand's, it's more likely that you've always had heavy bleeding during your periods. You may bruise easily, get nosebleeds, or bleeding gums; perhaps you've bled heavily after surgery or dental work.

Medical professionals strongly suggest that women with heavy bleeding be tested for these problems before agreeing to invasive procedures. A simple blood test can measure whether your blood clots normally.

IN A SENTENCE:

> Be able to rule out other problems before attributing common symptoms of those problems to fibroids.

DAY 5

living

Take a Look
Around Your Kitchen;
Take a Shopping Trip

TODAY MIGHT be a good day to do something practical
around the house. Let's go to the kitchen.

There are lots of reasons to believe that what we eat can
make a difference in how big our fibroids can get and how rap-
idly they can grow. Fibroids can grow in response to foods that
help create higher estrogen levels in our bodies, and they may
shrink in response to a diet that starves them of what they
crave.

Taking a look at the foods you eat and considering whether
you want to make changes can be a constructive thing to do
while you're getting used to having fibroids. Even if you decide
you're doing everything right in the diet department, understanding how food can affect your fibroids will help put you in
more control of your body and your health.

You don't have to change everything you eat, but it might be
interesting to take a look around your kitchen to see which of
your normal everyday foods should be eaten a little less often.

Let's start out by taking a kitchen inventory. After taking a close new look at your cabinets, cupboards, and refrigerator, you'll be able to write out a shopping list for your next trip to the grocery full of foods that can help your body fight fibroids.

These are a few of the common sources of **phytoestrogens** (literally, plant estrogens), fiber, and other healthy ingredients that can be a valuable part of your fibroid-fighting diet. How many of these things are in your kitchen right now?

- ❍ Soy foods, like tofu, tempeh, and soybeans
- ❍ High fiber breads and cereals
- ❍ Brown rice or other whole grains like barley and quinoa
- ❍ Red, green, and yellow vegetables, like tomatoes, peppers, and squash
- ❍ Root vegetables, like carrots and potatoes
- ❍ Fresh fruit, like apples and cherries
- ❍ Dried fruit, like dates and figs
- ❍ Canned or dried beans, like kidney beans, navy beans, and chick-peas

Now take a look to see which items in your kitchen contain these fibroid-friendly ingredients:

- ❍ Sugar
- ❍ Caffeine, in coffee, tea, sodas, and chocolate
- ❍ High fat foods, including pizza, fries, burgers, tacos
- ❍ Carbohydrates, especially food made with white flour, like white bread, pasta, cookies, and cakes
- ❍ Alcohol
- ❍ **Saturated fats**, found in animal products such as meat, chicken with the skin, eggs, and full-fat dairy products like cheese, ice cream, and butter. Coconut, palm, and cottonseed oils are the plant oils which are saturated.
- ❍ **Trans-fats**, found in partially hydrogenated oil, margarine, vegetable shortening, commercial baked goods, fried foods, many fast foods, most prepared snacks, mixes, and convenience foods.

Finding some of these ingredients in the foods you have in your kitchen may require looking at labels, especially on prepared foods, mixes, sodas, juice drinks, sweets, even bread, cereal, and crackers.

If you have time and energy, take your foods from the second list and put the bags, boxes, and bottles on the kitchen table. Now take a look at what's left in the cabinets and fridge. You'll see right away whether your diet—and your family's—veers toward fibroid-fighting (list 1) or fibroid friendly (list 2).

Many of the fibroid-friendly foods you have at home can be easily replaced with healthier alternatives. For instance, instead of buying white bread you can try whole wheat bread; instead of sweetened sodas you could try switching to flavored seltzer. Other foods may be harder to replace, like high-fat french fries or premium ice creams. You can decide whether to make big changes or start with small steps. Whichever you choose, your first stop is the market, where you can begin to stock your shelves for a fibroid-fighting diet.

Make a shopping list

If you want to try out some new or different foods, make a shopping list or bring this book with you when you go to the supermarket. As you go down the aisles, take a minute to notice where you find new or unfamiliar items on the list . . . this may help you remember where to find these items when you go back to the store without a list.

The vegetable aisle: Items here contain complex carbohydrates, fiber, phytoestrogens, vitamins, and minerals; some are also sources of healthy fats.

- Red, yellow, and green vegetables, like tomatoes, red peppers, and radishes; squash and yams; spinach, broccoli, kale, cabbage, cucumbers, green peppers, dandelion, celery, arugula, and swiss chard
- Other produce, like cauliflower, mushrooms, and eggplant
- Root vegetables, like carrots and potatoes
- Fresh fruit, like apples, cherries, pears, berries, citrus fruits, grapes, bananas, cantaloupes, and watermelon
- Dried fruit, like dates, figs, and apricots
- Seasonings, like garlic and ginger
- Nuts and seeds like walnuts, almonds, hazelnuts, macadamia nuts, and flaxseeds

The meat department: The right items here can help reduce your consumption of unhealthy fats and add minerals.

- ○ Fish, especially salmon and tuna, but also rainbow trout, mackerel, herring, sable, whitefish, eel, sardines, bluefish, swordfish, and haddock
- ○ Shellfish, like scallops, mussels, and clams
- ○ Wild game, such as rabbit and venison
- ○ Low fat cuts of chicken, veal, beef, or pork, preferably marked organic or steroid-free

The dairy case: Choices you make here can help you reduce your estrogen levels and lower your consumption of fat.

- ○ Soy foods, including tofu, tempeh, soy milk, soy ice cream, and soy yogurts
- ○ Non-fat dairy products, including milk, cheese, yogurt, and frozen desserts (best bet: look for labels that say "organic," or "we don't use bovine growth hormone [BGH]")
- ○ "Shelf milk," which doesn't require refrigeration
- ○ Non-dairy frozen desserts, such as all-natural sorbets
- ○ Sheep's cheese (such as feta or Romano), or goat cheese
- ○ Parmesan and mozzarella cheeses

The cooking and salad oil aisle: You can choose more healthful oils here.

- ○ Monounsaturated fats, found in olive, canola, sesame, and peanut oils, high-oleic sunflower seed oil, and high-oleic safflower seed oil
- ○ Omega-6 fatty acids, found in corn, safflower, sunflower, soybean, and sesame oils

The bread, grains, and bean aisles: Items found here can help you increase your intake of fiber.

- ○ High fiber breads and cereals
- ○ Oat bran
- ○ Brown rice or other whole grains like barley and quinoa
- ○ Beans, like kidney, navy, and chickpeas (dried or canned)

The beverage aisle: Make choices with less sugar; increase choices with vitamins and minerals.

○ If you drink soda or juice drinks, buy sugar-free varieties or flavored seltzer

○ Natural fruit juices, such as orange, tomato, and prune juice

The vitamin shelves: These can't replace the benefits of eating fresh, healthy foods, but taking the recommended daily amount can help your body fight fibroids. (Check with a doctor or nutritionist before adding unusual amounts of vitamins to your diet.)

○ Blue-green algae: Adds healthy Omega-6 fatty acids

○ Bioflavonoids: Replaces some of your natural estrogen with milder phytoestrogens

○ Black currant oil, evening primrose oil: Contain Gamma-linolenic acid (GLA); help decrease estrogen by controlling insulin levels

○ Flaxseed oil, fish oil supplements: add healthy Omega-3 fatty acids

○ I3C: Reduces estradiol, a strong form of estrogen

○ Lycopene: Reduces free radicals

○ Potassium: Helps prevent fibroid growth

○ Selenium: Strengthens immune system

○ Vitamins A, B Complex, C, E: Reduce free radicals

○ Zinc: Strengthens immune system

IN A SENTENCE:

> *Making smart choices about food can help you fight fibroids.*

learning

What Foods Can Help/Hurt and Why

YOU ALREADY know the old joke that chocolate goes directly to your hips . . . but deep in your heart you know that something chemical has to happen in between. It's the same with fibroids: While foods don't literally feed your fibroids, they still may affect how fast fibroids grow. Why?

○ Certain foods affect the estrogen levels in your blood, and estrogen can be a factor in how your fibroids grow.

○ Body fat helps convert **androgens**, male hormones we have in small amounts, into estrogen. The more body fat we have, the more of this conversion takes place and the more our risk for fibroids increases.

○ Too much fat, sugar, and other common foods may put stress on your liver. Since the liver is what processes extra estrogen out of our bodies, it makes sense to make its job as easy as possible.

The benefits of fibroid-fighting foods

One of the goals of a fibroid-fighting diet is to help regulate the amount of estrogen in our systems. At least 300 plants—soy in particular—have phytoestrogens (literally, plant estrogens), also called bioflavonoids and isoflavones. Phytoestrogens are much weaker than our natural estrogen or even synthetic estrogens, but they have a similar chemical structure, so they can block the absorption of "real" estrogen into our systems, helping to reduce estrogen-related problems we may have.

Can phytoestrogens help reduce our fibroids? The answer depends on your stage of life.

Before **perimenopause**, phytoestrogens can help reduce the amount of estrogen in our systems by blocking access to some estrogen receptors; since the "real" estrogen can't get into the blocked receptors, our overall estrogen levels go down. As a result, there may be less estrogen available to feed our fibroids.

In perimenopause, estrogen levels fluctuate much more than usual, and declining progesterone may make the effect much more pronounced. By experimenting with phytoestrogen-rich foods, you may be able to tone down the effects of all those "power surges"—and help reduce or prevent growth spurts in your fibroids.

On the other hand, it is possible to overdo it. Even though phytoestrogens are natural, too much can have unintended effects. If you stick to phytoestrogens in food form, such as soy, you'd pretty much have to eat all phyto all the time to hurt your system, but supplements and herbs can be very potent and should only be taken after consulting with a qualified nutritionist, **naturopath**, **homeopath**, or doctor of Chinese medicine.

Once you've reached menopause, and the amount of natural estrogen in your system is waning, phytoestrogens can provide a mild form of estrogen. On the other hand, if you're on Hormone Replacement Therapy (HRT), too many phytoestrogens can block the effect. The same cautions about working with a qualified health care practitioner apply for any herbs or supplements you'd like to explore at this stage of life. In either case, talk to your doctor about whether you should monitor your fibroids on a regular basis.

Soy

Of all the plants that produce phytoestrogens, soy may have the most protective effect. In particular, Dr. Susan Lark tells us that soy has been found to help reduce bleeding problems in women with fibroids. This may be because soy foods include a substance called genistein that, in tests, blocked the growth of new blood vessels.

If you decide to eat soy for its protective benefits, it's important to be consistent, making soy products a part of your daily diet. How can you do that? Studies suggest that you can get adequate amounts of phytoestrogens by drinking four glasses of soy milk a day or a drink made from soy-protein powder. Other sources include tofu, tempeh, and miso, or you could try soy burgers (veggie burgers) or even soy hotdogs, soy-based cheese, soy ice cream, and soy yogurts. To get the protective benefits of soy, doctors recommend eating or drinking 40 grams of soy protein a day.

FIBER

Dietary fiber—from 15 to 30 grams per day—can reduce blood estrogen levels, one of the things that may help fibroids grow. Fiber isn't that hard to find: apples have lots of fiber, as do just about every other fruit, most veggies, whole grains like brown rice, whole wheat, and old-fashioned oatmeal, nuts, and seeds.

How does it work? Dietary fiber speeds waste products through our bodies. If waste sits in our intestines, the accumulated toxins sit there too, and some of them get reabsorbed through our intestinal walls. Fiber picks up all those toxins, including fats, and gives them a quicker ride out of your body. (As a result, fiber can also help relieve constipation, a problem that affects up to half of all women with fibroids.)

An important counterpart to eating more fiber is drinking more water. At least eight glasses of clear uncarbonated water a day will help your body detoxify.

VEGGIES

Vegetables are a major source of almost all the vitamins, minerals, and natural chemicals that may play a role in helping control fibroid growth and symptoms. As we saw in our shopping list, an easy way to remember much of what you need is to think in color: yellow, red, and green.

Yellow and gold vegetables like carrots, butternut squash, and yams, just to name a few, contain the powerful **beta-carotenes**, which protect us against free radicals. Free radicals are molecules which trigger cell abnormalities, possibly including fibroids. Dark green leafy veggies like spinach and kale are also good sources of beta-carotenes.

Broccoli, arugula, cabbage, kale, and other dark green vegetables include something called **Indole-3 carbinol** (I3C), a chemical that does two things:

it prevents the development of cells that respond to estrogen, and converts estradiol, a powerful form of estrogen, into the milder form called estrone.

Like tomatoes? The same substance that turns tomatoes red can help reduce the free radicals in your system, even more powerfully than the beta-carotenes.

Fruits are also nutritional treasure troves. Watermelon, mango, cherries, and the whole rainbow of brightly colored fruits help provide healthful protection against free radicals. The only thing to remember as you work out a balanced diet is that fruit contains more sugar than vegetables, and as we'll see in a moment, sugar is something we should all try to limit in our diets.

How fibroid-friendly foods can increase fibroid growth

As we discussed, certain foods can have a negative effect on your fibroids, although the effects may be indirect. None of these products will kill us, but if you eat a lot of the following types of foods, you might want to consider putting them on your "buy less often" list, while substituting more healthful alternatives.

MEAT AND POULTRY

You may already know that meat and poultry with high levels of saturated fat can raise your cholesterol levels; this includes fatty cuts of beef, pork, or veal, and chicken or turkey cooked with the skin on. Cholesterol can get converted to estrogen in our bodies . . . which can result in fibroid growth, heavier bleeding, and other symptoms.

Meat that includes high levels of saturated fat can also be stressful on the liver. If your liver is overworked, it is less able to break down estrogen—resulting in more estrogen circulating in your bloodstream. Once again, this can lead to fibroid growth, heavier bleeding, cramps, or pressure.

In addition to the natural properties of fatty meats, many animals raised for food, especially in the United States, are treated with drugs called **anabolic steroids** to make them bigger and heavier, providing more meat per animal.

The Food and Drug Administration (FDA) maintains that the level of drugs used is no threat to humans—even children. However, some scientists tell us that when animals ingest antibiotics, pesticides, or growth hormones, these substances accumulate in the animal's fat. If we eat treated animals, the fat in our own bodies accumulates and stores these sub-stances, where they can stay for as long as twenty years. These substances may raise your estrogen levels—which in turn may lead to fibroid growth and symptoms.

We do need protein, and not all of us are cut out to be vegetarians. If you don't want to stop eating meat, consider cutting down. These three tips will also help:

○ Select lean meat or skinless poultry.
○ Broil or grill to well-done to help cook out remaining fat, and don't use the drippings.
○ Look for organically raised meat to avoid the steroids that may be present in commercially-raised meat.

DAIRY

Like high fat meat, full-fat dairy products contribute to raising your cho-lesterol levels and making your liver work overtime. In addition, the fat in dairy products contains **arachidonic acid**; this stimulates our bodies to pro-duce prostaglandins, which can cause pelvic pain and cramps. For this rea-son, both Dr. Christiane Northrup and Dr. Susan Lark advise women with fibroids to avoid dairy products made from cow's milk, since they can lead to higher levels of both estrogen and prostaglandins.

Again, apart from the natural properties of cow's milk, artificial hor-mones may be an issue. About one-third of U.S. dairy cattle are given some-thing called **bovine growth hormone** (BGH) to increase milk production. Unfortunately, BGH produces a hormone called **insulinlike growth fac-tor-1** (IGF-1), which may have a role in fibroid growth, as well as in prostate cancer and breast cancer.

According to the FDA, milk from treated cows is safe for human con-sumption; as a result, products made from BGH-treated cows' milk aren't labeled as such. However, Canadian researchers found that BGH was absorbed into the bloodstream of almost a third of the animals studied in lab tests. So until dairy food producers start including BGH on their labels, consider buying organic milk products.

You don't have to cut down or give up every kind of dairy food: Nonfat yogurt, cheese, and milk products are safe bets because they don't contain arachidonic acid. Small quantities of Parmesan, mozzarella, or shelf milk are fine, as are sheep's cheese (such as feta or Romano) and goat cheese or yogurt.

FAT

Fat can affect fibroids in four negative ways:

1. Fat from animal products may store toxins or extra hormones that can be transferred to your body.
2. Fat can raise cholesterol levels; cholesterol can convert into estrogen, raising your overall estrogen levels.
3. Saturated and polyunsaturated fats are easily oxidized into "free radicals," which may potentially weaken your immune system.
4. Omega-6 and trans-fats produce prostaglandins, which can cause cramps.

Choosing your fats wisely can help control your fibroid growth or symptoms. Of all the fats we can eat, saturated and trans-fats are the ones to really consider minimizing. These are the fats hardest to resist, showing up as they do in fries, pizza, tacos, ice cream, cheese, and every kind of meat and chicken . . . but if you want to reduce your intake of these fats, keep these foods to a minimum, check labels, avoid deep-fried foods, and choose skim or fat-free dairy products.

SUGAR

One of the easiest things to spot in your diet are foods containing sugar. There's candy, of course, along with cookies, cakes, sweetened cereals, and other treats. However, there's also sugar in many prepackaged foods and mixes, or more subtly, in carbohydrates such as bread, pasta, potatoes, rice, and fruit.

Whether it's in candy bars or corn muffins, too much sugar may take its toll on us and our fibroids in five ways:

1. First, by raising insulin levels. Extra insulin decreases **sex hormone binding globulin** (SHBG). Since SHBG binds free estrogen, less SHBG means that more estrogen is circulating in your bloodstream.
2. Extra insulin has been traditionally associated with weight gain; extra body fat may increase your circulating estrogen.

3. Sugar reduces vitamin B, which can make it harder for your liver to process estrogen out of your system.
4. Sugar depletes our bodies of the nutrients needed to keep our immune systems intact.
5. Even relying on sugar substitutes may not be the answer: consumer groups have raised questions about aspartame, the ingredient in popular sugar substitutes, which some studies have linked to increased incidence of tumors in the uterus as well as the brain and pancreas.

If you want to consider reducing the amount of sugar in your diet, here are a few suggestions:

○ think about reducing or eliminating refined sugar, the kind in candy, cookies, and other desserts;
○ remember that there's a lot of sugar in regular soda, regular fruit juice, juice drinks, and presweetened tea and coffee;
○ consider cutting back on white flour products in favor of whole-grain foods;
○ when you eat complex carbohydrates, try eating them along with some protein and vegetables. According to Dr. Andrew Weil, eating carbohydrates as part of a balanced meal slows down insulin production;
○ if sugary foods are your "comfort food" when you're stressed or sad, maybe you can pick out a healthier alternative—and have it in the kitchen for when those cravings hit;
○ and if by any chance you need another incentive to exercise, it can help keep your insulin levels in check.

CAFFEINE AND ALCOHOL

While caffeine doesn't seem to be directly related to fibroids, there are a few indirect ways that caffeine may have an impact on fibroid-related symptoms:

○ Drinking a lot of caffeine can interfere with how well your liver functions; it can also aggravate fibroid-related cramps.
○ Drinking coffee or tea after eating can reduce the amount of iron your body can absorb, which is important to know if you're anemic.

○ A recent study showed that drinking 4–5 cups of coffee a day can increase your stress levels: we'll talk about why this is an important issue for your fibroids in Month 2.

Green tea contains some caffeine, but there's more and more evidence piling up that it has a number of general health benefits. Herbal teas don't contain caffeine.

Alcohol is another beverage that may have an indirect effect on fibroids. Most of us know that alcohol is bad for the liver, and being kind to your liver, as we've seen, is a key component in keeping your estrogen levels down. If your fibroids are causing cramps, fatigue, or bleeding, alcohol can make them worse. If your fibroids aren't bothering you, enjoying an occasional drink shouldn't hurt as long as it's part of a generally healthful diet.

IN A SENTENCE:

Moderating your diet can help strengthen your body and immune system, and may help inhibit fibroid growth.

Stop By the Drugstore;
The Natural Foods Store

YESTERDAY WE worked on the kitchen. Today, let's turn our attention to the medicine cabinet. Our objective today is to put together a "Symptoms Survival Kit." This means making sure you have all the items on hand you might need to soothe your fibroid symptoms, from menstrual cramps to tension headaches. If you don't have the things you need in the house already, you can get them quickly and easily at the neighborhood drugstore and natural foods store.

Your Symptoms Survival Kit shouldn't replace regular doctor's visits, and if your symptoms are severe or recurring, you may need more extensive treatments that only doctors or other medical professionals can provide. But a home Symptoms Survival Kit can be the first line of defense against the day-to-day problems that fibroids can provoke.

There are four steps to creating your Symptoms Survival Kit:

○ First, you'll need to take stock of the symptoms that are bothering you. On Day 3, you started a diary to keep track of your symptoms. (If you haven't started it yet, why not grab a piece of paper and begin now?) Take a look at what you wrote down. Are you bleeding heavily? Have cramps? Are you constipated? Are you feeling panicky or upset?

○ Second, decide on a handy place to keep everything. You might want to choose a deep basket or plastic milk crate that you can keep in your bathroom, kitchen, or bedroom. Items needing refrigeration can be placed in a plastic container in the fridge. It's important to know what you have and where you have it, so you can reach it quickly and easily as soon as you want it. Of course, if you have small children, the items in your Symptoms Survival Kit should be kept out of reach.

○ Third, we'll take a look at what you might want in your kit, depending on your symptoms. You may find that you already have many of these items in your medicine cabinet or kitchen.

○ Fourth, you'll want to do a little shopping to fill in whatever items you don't already have.

If you don't already have the following items at home, here's a shopping list to help you create your Symptoms Survival Kit.

At the drugstore
○ Over the counter pain remedies: aspirin, **ibuprofen,** or **naproxen**
○ Sanitary pads (instead of or in addition to tampons)
○ Hot water bottle or heating pad
○ Vitamins and minerals specific to fibroid symptoms:
- Beta-carotenes
- Calcium
- Iron
- Linolenic acid
- Magnesium
- Potassium
- Vitamin B_6
- Vitamin C
- Vitamin E

Natural foods store
○ Fresh ginger root
○ Castor oil (optional)

○ Essential oils:
  - One or more of the following: chamomile, lavender, marjoram, melissa
  - One or both of the following: rose or jasmine
○ Unscented massage or bath oil, like apricot seed or grapeseed oil
○ Herbal teas: ginger, cinnamon, or peppermint
○ Flaxseed
○ Valerian root capsules

When you bring these items home, mark the bottles and boxes with a bright adhesive label or magic marker so you can identify them easily.

IN A SENTENCE:

> *Assemble a Symptoms Survival Kit from items at the drugstore and natural foods store.*

learning

How These Remedies Work

If you have cramps

There are more simple remedies for cramps than for any other symptom. Here are the hows and whys of the items that can go in your Symptoms Survival Kit.

Over-the-counter pain remedies. Aspirin and the drugs known generically as ibuprofen and naproxen can help control cramps and bleeding by either slowing down the production of prostaglandins, or by actually lowering estrogen levels. Of course, if you have very painful cramps or heavy bleeding, or want to take more than the recommended doses of any medicine, talk to your doctor.

Sanitary pads instead of tampons can prevent potential irritation leading to cramps.

Gentle heat can relax tense abdominal muscles and ease the pain of cramps. There are a few different ways to bring heat to your belly:

○ Heating pad or hot water bottle, placed on your abdomen or back when cramps are troubling you.

○ Castor oil packs may help soothe menstrual cramps. Different sources recommend using a castor oil pack for about half an hour once a day, or at least once a week.

- What you need: castor oil, preferably from a health food store; a large towel or sheet to protect your bed, couch, or carpet from spilled oil; a warm cloth, like flannel; hot water bottle or heating pad.
- What to do: Spread out the towel or sheet; lie down on top of it. Using a bath sponge or your fingers, spread castor oil over your abdomen. Put the warm cloth over the castor oil; put a hot water bottle or heating pad over the cloth.
- If you want, add a quarter teaspoon of scented essential oil to the castor oil before you spread it on; you can also warm the flannel in the dryer before you use it, or gently warm the castor oil in a pot on top of the stove before use—make sure it's warm but not hot, so that you don't burn yourself.

○ You can make a similar compress with fresh ginger tea.

- What you'll need: fresh ginger root, peeled and chopped into small chunks; hot water; a flannel cloth.
- What to do: Place the cut ginger in a bowl or pot and pour boiling water over it; cover and let the mixture steep for about ten minutes.
- Make sure the tea is hot but comfortable; soak your flannel cloth in the tea, wring it out, and place it on your abdomen. You can put a hot water bottle over the wet cloth if you like—but not an electric heating pad.

○ A warm bath. You don't need anything special, but if you like, you can add a few drops of essential oil: chamomile, lavender, marjoram, and melissa are all scents thought to relieve cramps; rose and jasmine are thought to be good for uterine disorders. (Don't use water that's too hot to sit in comfortably, or do this if you have high blood pressure, a heart condition, or are pregnant.)

○ Herbal teas can warm you from the inside out. Certain types may also soothe cramps; try ginger, cinnamon, or peppermint. (As above, you can make your own herbal teas by placing fresh sliced ginger, a cinnamon stick, or a small bunch of peppermint leaves in a teapot.

Pour boiling water over them, let the tea steep for several minutes, and strain before drinking.)

Vitamins. Certain vitamins and minerals can help with some of the symptoms you may have, including cramps.

In general, if you can get your vitamins and minerals from food, they'll be more effective. But since eating a balanced diet is more a goal than a reality for many of us, you may choose to take some supplements.

Remember, don't take more than the recommended amount without consulting a doctor or nutritionist. Excess amounts of some vitamins or minerals can be counter-productive or even toxic, depending on your diet, certain allergies, and other medical conditions, so please, consult your doctor or a trained nutritionist about the right amounts to include in your diet. Also ask if he or she can recommend a brand or brands of supplements. Since these so-called "nutraceuticals" aren't regulated, quality control varies widely.

Here are the vitamins and minerals that can help relieve cramps, along with common food sources:

- ○ Calcium (also found in dairy products, collard greens, canned salmon, and sardines with the bones)
- ○ Magnesium (also found in kale, collard, chard, watercress, whole grains, beans, nuts, seeds, fruit, chicken, seafood, potatoes)
- ○ Potassium (also found in bananas, oranges, cantaloupes, spinach, potatoes, bran flakes, prune juice, tomato juice)
- ○ Vitamin B_6 (also found in meat, grains, beans, bananas, leafy green vegetables, corn, peas, nuts, fish, garlic)
- ○ Vitamin C (also found in citrus fruits, broccoli, leafy green vegetables, tomatoes, peppers, strawberries, cantaloupe, potatoes)
- ○ Vitamin E (also found in wheat germ, oatmeal, nuts, brown rice, soy, asparagus, cabbage, leafy green vegetables). If you are bleeding heavily, you should not take extra vitamin E, since it can slow down the coagulation of blood.
- ○ Linolenic acid (also found in many fruits and vegetables, flaxseeds)

In addition, the herb valerian, which is most commonly known for its sleep-inducing properties, is also thought to relieve cramps.

If you're bleeding heavily

Unfortunately, there are few home remedies for heavy bleeding. Still, there are a few items you should be sure to have in your Symptoms Survival Kit:

Sanitary pads to supplement tampons in case of heavy bleeding or flooding. Women who bleed heavily advise you to have lots of pads on hand.

Vitamins. Several vitamins and minerals may help relieve bleeding, or add iron to help prevent anemia. Again, don't take more than the recommended amount of each supplement without consulting a doctor or nutritionist.

- O Beta-carotenes (also found in carrots, squash, yams, cantaloupe, bok choy, sweet potatoes, apricots, spinach, corn, kale, turnip greens, citrus fruits)
- O Iron (also found in beef, lamb, pork, turkey, chicken, beans, soy, whole grains, dried fruit, dark green leafy vegetables, black cherries, dandelion, celery, parsley, seaweed, and by cooking in iron pots)
- O Vitamin C (also found in citrus fruits, broccoli, leafy green vegetables, tomatoes, peppers, strawberries, cantaloupe, potatoes)

If you feel bloated, or have constipation

Flaxseed: Sprinkle up to three teaspoons of flaxseed (available at health food stores) on food every day: perhaps on top of cereal, or in a salad. It's a healthy and simple remedy that seems to relieve bloating, aid digestion, and help reduce fibroid growth.

If you just want to relax

Essential oils/aromatherapy scents: rose, jasmine, chamomile, and lavender are all relaxing. Put a few drops of the essential oil of your choice in an ounce of unscented oil, like apricot seed or grapeseed oil, before adding to your bath or using for massage; remember, essential oils are for external use only. Use caution with essential oils if you're pregnant.

There's one other category of items you might want to include in your Symptoms Survival Kit: a few things that will remind you to take time out to relax when the stress of having fibroids threatens to get to you. Include anything you like—a favorite book of poems, a soothing CD or cassette, a copy of *Young Frankenstein* for laughs. Don't forget to include a couple of treats like raspberry bubble bath and a small scented candle for a sweet-smelling candlelit bath.

IN A SENTENCE:

Items in your Symptoms Survival Kit can help ease cramps, make bleeding more manageable, and help you deal with stress.

Setting Up an Exercise Schedule

IT'S BEEN a long week. You've been through a lot and done a lot of work. While you've been getting used to the idea of having fibroids, and letting that reality settle in, you've also been working, taking care of your home, and doing all of the other things that filled up your days before you ever heard of fibroids.

So take a deep breath and congratulate yourself for getting through Week 1. Just by taking the first step of getting informed and getting ideas about how to manage your fibroids, you've made the important decision to take control of your life and control your fibroids, rather than let them control you. Now comes your next job.

You don't need me to tell you about the benefits of exercising. If you already have an exercise program, you're ahead of the game. If not, your fibroids can provide one more incentive to start working out.

If you're a real novice, use today to start something gentle. Take a ten-minute walk, borrow your teenager's bicycle and take a ride, or try doing some stretching. Most importantly, mark your calendar: decide right now which days and times of the week you can dedicate to a half hour of exercise, and plan on sticking with it. It's hard to fit in, I know, but consider

○ using half of your lunch hour at work to take a walk;
○ renting an exercise video to do in the morning;
○ signing up for a group class in beginners' yoga, tai chi, Latin dance, or whatever you've been telling yourself you would do "one of these days."

In addition to exercising three times a week, or more, you can also sneak some extra minutes in by taking the dog out for a walk in the evening, making extra trips up and down the stairs at home, or taking a bike ride on the weekend.

If you already belong to a gym and don't go as often as you planned, or if you have an exercise hobby that you once enjoyed, use today to re-commit. What type of exercise can you commit to, how many times a week, for how long? Be realistic as you start out: plan on a shorter amount of time in the beginning just to get back in the habit and keep yourself from getting too tired or too discouraged.

Take a look at the list on the next page and fill in your commitment—to yourself. Then take out your day planner or calendar and write down exactly which days and times you plan to exercise. Write in your appointments to exercise for at least the next month. It will be easier to follow through if you already have the time booked in your schedule. Make a date with a buddy—someone you enlisted earlier for your Fibroid Support Team—to try something new.

Don't put it off. Start by going for a walk, run, or ride, right now.

IN A SENTENCE:

> *Re-commit to exercise to help fight your fibroids.*

MY EXERCISE COMMITMENT

Type of exercise I commit to	Times per week	Minutes per day
Walking	_____	_____
Biking	_____	_____
Swimming	_____	_____
Jogging	_____	_____
Treadmill	_____	_____
Yoga	_____	_____
Light weights	_____	_____
Dance	_____	_____
Martial Arts	_____	_____
Tai chi	_____	_____
Other	_____	_____

learning

Benefits of Exercise

THE BENEFITS of exercise are well-known. Optimal amounts of time to spend exercising vary with each new report, but the minimum requirement to stay healthy seems to be thirty minutes, five to six times a week.

It's always wise to check with your doctor before starting a new exercise program. It's also a good idea to start slow and work up to your desired time and intensity level. Steady, moderate exercise has a number of benefits, helping you fight your fibroids at least five ways:

1. Weight loss: Body fat helps increase the amount of estrogen in our systems; as we'll see more in the next chapter, estrogen is a major culprit in the growth of fibroids.

2. Reduces cholesterol: Circulating cholesterol can convert to estrogen.

3. Helps control insulin: Correct amounts of insulin in your system help regulate proper estrogen levels. Too much insulin has been traditionally associated with weight gain.

4. Relieves mild symptoms: Light aerobic exercise, even a walk around the block, can help relieve painful cramps

by increasing your circulation, relaxing your muscles, and releasing pain-killing beta-endorphins.

5. Relieves stress: Stress may release stored toxins in our bodies, which may also affect estrogen levels.

IN A SENTENCE:

> *As if you needed one more reason to work out, regular exercise can also help control the growth of your fibroids, and fibroid symptoms.*

FIRST-WEEK MILESTONE

By the end of your first week you've taken the first crucial steps to taking control of your fibroids, as you have now:

○ LEARNED WHAT FIBROIDS ARE, AND WHAT CAUSES THEM.

○ NOMINATED A FIBROID SUPPORT TEAM TO HELP YOU GET THE SUPPORT YOU NEED FROM FAMILY AND FRIENDS.

○ STARTED A LIFESTYLE AND SYMPTOMS INDICATOR TO HELP MAKE CONNECTIONS BETWEEN YOUR LIFESTYLE HABITS AND YOUR FIBROID SYMPTOMS.

○ STARTED SHOPPING FOR HEALTHIER FOODS THAT CAN HELP YOUR BODY FIGHT FIBROIDS.

○ ASSEMBLED A HOME SYMPTOMS SURVIVAL KIT.

○ BEGUN OR RE-COMMITTED TO AN EXERCISE PROGRAM.

Keeping Track
of Your Period

IF YOU remember all the way back to Day 3, we talked about setting up a Lifestyle and Symptoms Indicator. Perhaps you've already seen that writing things down helps change your view of the world. It's the same thing with any aspect of your daily life; keeping a record of things that happen can give you a truer perspective on how what you do—and what happens to you—can affect you.

For the Lifestyle and Symptoms Indicator, we talked about keeping track of things that you do and have control over, like your diet, exercise program, and herbal medications you choose to take and their relationship to any symptoms you might have.

It's also important to keep a record of what your body is doing, in ways that you don't necessarily have control over. Most significantly, this means keeping track of your monthly period.

Think about it. Are your periods light, medium, or heavy, or do they change from month to month? Can you say with any certainty how many days your average period lasts, or how long a time it is between periods? Do you know when your symptoms, if any, occur in your cycle, or how severe your symptoms are month to month?

Now is your chance.

Today, we're going to add another element to your fibroid-management program: a Menstrual Period Diary. Your diary can be an important tool to help you and your doctor evaluate your symptoms. If you're experiencing any kind of unusual bleeding, you can use your diary to keep track of how frequently and how heavily you're bleeding. Adding your Menstrual Period Diary to your Lifestyle and Symptoms Indicator can help you pinpoint anything that might have triggered the bleeding to start, and any other symptoms, such as pain, fever, or changes in bowel or bladder function. Just to give one example, sometimes a combination of medications can influence bleeding: for instance, taking both aspirin and Ginkgo biloba may play a role in heavy bleeding.

Here are the items to track for your Menstrual Period Diary:

Day your most recent period began:	*[date]*
How many days it lasted:	*Example: 4 days*
Days since your last period began:	*Example: 28 days*
Big changes from last period:	*Lighter, heavier, or about the same*
Symptoms:	*Example: Heavy bleeding (and/or pain, fatigue, etc.)*
Severity:	*Mild, moderate, severe*
Frequency:	*Example: hourly cramps; for bleeding, how often pads and or tampons are changed*

If you're experiencing strong symptoms, it's helpful to track these day by day on your calendar: over time, patterns can emerge related to your menstrual cycle that can give you and your doctor important clues about the cause of your symptoms.

Why do you need to track this extra information in your Menstrual Period Diary?

○ You'll have a real-time record to share with your doctor that can help determine the kinds of treatment she recommends.
○ You'll be able to track the effectiveness of any natural or alternative treatments you choose to try.

○ You won't have to trust your memory or your feelings about what's going on; you'll have a realistic idea of how your fibroids are affecting you, how often you feel symptoms, and how severe you judge them to be.

IN A SENTENCE:

> *A Menstrual Period Diary can give you an accurate record of your periods and your fibroid symptoms and how the actions you take affect them.*

learning

The Role of Estrogen and Progesterone

ESTROGEN IS produced naturally in your body, by the ovaries and adrenal glands, but there are more than twenty different variations. The three major forms of estrogen your body produces are called:

- ○ **estradiol**, produced in the menstrual years by the ovaries, is the most powerful;
- ○ **estriol** reaches high levels during pregnancy;
- ○ **estrone**, made by fat cells, becomes the dominant estrogen after menopause, but can also add estrogen to your system while you're still menstruating. The heavier you are, the more estrone you produce.

Studies suggest that there are dramatic variations in "normal" estrogen between women. It seems logical to assume that these variations may account for the wide range of effects, both positive and negative, reported by women taking any type of hormone therapy, including the birth control pill, HRT, and **nutraceuticals** such as soy. (There may also be more of a distinction between the three major forms of estrogen than we currently imagine. A study which examined the presence of the three major types of estrogen [estradiol, estriol, and estrone] in a small group of women found that levels of estriol, often called the "weakest" of the three forms of estrogen in our systems, was often higher than estrone and estradiol combined. How the three types of estrogen interact, what the significance of high estrone levels are, and how these affect fibroids are all unknown; however, it is a sure bet that the eventual findings will show us a female hormonal system even more complex and delicate than we now know it to be.)

Estrogen plays a powerful part in keeping various parts of our bodies running smoothly, including our hearts, brains, and blood vessels. It helps us maintain healthy teeth, gums, bones, skin, and hair and increases blood flow to the vagina, creating more elasticity and lubrication. Estrogen may help reduce anxiety and depression, and even help maintain normal sleep cycles. Ironically, estrogen is also one of the key factors in the growth and development of fibroids.

Before menopause, estrogen and its sister hormone, progesterone, play a key role in our monthly periods. The production of estrogen and progesterone start, of all places, in our brains. Each month, when your period is over, your levels of estrogen and progesterone are at their lowest. Your **hypothalamus**, the "central command" in your brain, senses that it's time to start a new cycle and starts raising your estrogen levels again.

As your estrogen starts increasing, arteries in your uterine lining start growing. This is called **angiogenesis**, the creation of new blood vessels. These new blood vessels build up a layer of fresh blood in the uterus, making the lining up to three times thicker.

Just before mid-cycle, one of your ovaries releases an egg; this signals your body to begin making progesterone. When the egg completes its journey through the Fallopian tube and reaches the uterus, you're at mid-cycle, and at the height of your potential fertility.

What happens next depends on conception. If the egg is fertilized, you continue to make progesterone and your estrogen levels stay high. If the egg isn't fertilized, your body stops making progesterone and your estrogen levels go down. Without the high level of hormones to support it, the lining of the uterus falls away and blood flows freely into the cavity. This produces what we see as our monthly period.

At this point, you produce yet another hormone, called a prostaglandin, which makes the uterus contract. The contractions help push out the lining and squeeze the blood vessels in the uterus shut.

For women with fibroids, the natural fluctuations that start happening in our thirties or forties can have a big impact on fibroid growth and symptoms. In the years between youth and menopause, changes in estrogen levels can make our fibroids go through surprising growth spurts.

As we get a bit older, the ovaries need more stimulation to produce an egg each month. In response, the brain sends out extra amounts of a chemical called **follicle-stimulating hormone** (FSH). The extra FSH gets the ovaries to produce more estrogen than usual; higher levels of both FSH and estrogen can make your fibroids grow bigger. You also may get more bleeding, since estrogen stimulates blood flow to the uterus and FSH dilates blood vessels.

Around the same time of life, progesterone levels gradually start to go down. Since this generally starts happening while your estrogen levels are still high, your body has an imbalance of estrogen to progesterone; this leads to more of what doctors call "unopposed" estrogen, which can further fuel those fibroids.

Estrogen is absorbed into our bodies by **receptors**, special gateways into our cells. Certain substances can fool the receptors into thinking they're accepting our own natural estrogen when in fact they are not. These other substances may be potentially good for us or potentially toxic, and include:

○ phytoestrogens, which as we discussed on Day 5, are a form of estrogen that exists in plants.
○ medical synthetics, such as those used in Hormone Replacement Therapy (see Month 4 for more information about medical synthetics).
○ **xenoestrogens**, man-made compounds that appear in pesticides and other chemicals.

Xenoestrogens (pronounced "ZEE-no estrogens") are particularly troubling. They are very pervasive: According to the World Wildlife Fund, there are over 100,000 man-made chemicals used in virtually every industry, everywhere in the world. Of these, scientists agree that many are endocrine disrupters or xenoestrogens (meaning "foreign estrogens").

Scientists have been raising warnings about xenoestrogens and their effects on women, including the risk of fibroids, since at least 1993. In testimony before the Senate Committee on Labor and Human Resources, government scientists confirmed that these environmental compounds may play a role in the growth of fibroids and a wide range of other diseases, including cancers of the breast, uterus, and ovaries.

Two new studies, called TULEP and BULB, are being funded by the National Institute of Child Health and Human Development; the goal of the studies is to determine the relationship between fibroids and different types of estrogen, including those found in food, the environment, and medicines. Look for the results of these studies in the near future.

Here's how chemical estrogens can affect our bodies and our fibroids:

O Since they are stored in our bodies, chemical estrogens can be released at any time, often when we're under stress, or even when we diet. Tests show that some of these chemicals can spur dramatic growth of uterine cells or increase cell division.

O Some chemical estrogens make our bodies produce more estradiol, the strongest type of natural estrogen, raising our natural estrogen levels.

O Some of these chemicals depress thyroid hormone function; a healthy thyroid is essential to helping the liver process estrogen out of our bodies.

O Some may permanently alter our DNA; this effect may be passed down to our daughters—and granddaughters.

For many of us, chemical pesticides may be the single worst form of xenoestrogens. Pesticides are most often found on both the foods we eat and the outdoor spaces we use (public parks, golf courses, and so on). Simple actions, like thoroughly washing fruits, vegetables, and fresh herbs, buying organic foods when possible, using organic pesticides at home, and making sure everyone in the family washes their hands carefully when they come inside, can all help reduce your family's risk for consuming xenoestrogens.

Progesterone

Progesterone, as we saw, is a hormone that works in partnership with estrogen to regulate pregnancy and our periods. If your body is not making enough progesterone to balance your estrogen, unchecked estrogen may contribute to helping fibroids grow. Similarly, it's possible that high levels of progesterone may also be a factor in fibroid growth.

Progesterone appears to stimulate a hormone called **vascular endothelial growth factor (VEGF)**, which helps create blood vessels that can feed both normal cells and tumors. Since fibroids are dependent on blood to feed them, more VEGF in your system could help make your fibroids grow faster. Estrogen may help regulate VEGF; once again, it seems possible that the problem is not estrogen or progesterone in themselves, but when your body begins to have an imbalance of one or the other.

Scientists are studying how **antiprogesterones** (also called **antiprogestins**) can be used to develop new treatments for fibroids. Unfortunately, even though doctors regard antiprogesterones as safe, everyday use of them to treat fibroids is unlikely in the United States anytime soon— since an antiprogesterone called mifepristone is the key ingredient in RU-486, the so-called abortion pill. The controversy over using RU-486 to induce abortions has overshadowed its other medical uses, including fibroid treatment. However, doctors may be able to prescribe "off-label" use of mifepristone for fibroids. See Month 4 for more on mifepristone as well as off-label prescribing.

Fortunately, Congress has not prohibited the NIH from conducting or supporting research on mifepristone and other antiprogestins in hopes of developing treatments for fibroid tumors, amoung other reproductive diseases. (Research on mifepristone as an abortion agent is currently restricted.)

IN A SENTENCE:

> *Estrogen and progesterone are complex hormones that may have the most effect on our fibroids when they are out of balance with each other.*

Considering Natural Progestrone

NATURAL PROGESTERONE, made from wild yam, is offered by a variety of manufacturers as a cure for fibroid symptoms, among other claims. The Canadian government banned the sale of progesterone creams in 1997 since the manufacturers could not offer enough proof that their products worked as claimed. In the United States, the FDA approves natural progesterone for oral consumption, but creams are unregulated. Natural progesterone cream was originally offered as a way to prevent osteoporosis; sources are extremely mixed as to how well—or if—progesterone cream works on fibroids. One recent study concluded that a skin cream made from wild yam had no more effect on women's hormones than a **placebo**.

Despite this, some women do find that natural progesterone cream can help relieve symptoms like heavy bleeding and severe PMS. It's possible that the women who find relief are those whose estrogen levels are surging while their progesterone levels are declining. However, until studies can show consistently that natural progesterone cream relieves fibroid symptoms, we can only speculate.

WEEK **3**

living

What Does Having Fibroids Mean to You?

LATER IN this chapter we'll start to go over your treatment options, which are actually becoming more numerous all the time. But before you can begin to decide on treatment, if any, it's important to put your fibroids in context. What are your life plans and how might your fibroids affect those plans?

Unless your symptoms are extreme, you have time to think about your treatment choices, do your homework, talk to women who've made the choice or choices you're investigating. But remember, you're unique; no one else has your physical, emotional, or sexual concerns. No one else has your specific lifestyle situation or goals. It's important to take the time to think about who you are, what you want, and the impact of any treatments you're considering.

First of all, you should take a moment to even consider whether your fibroids are bothering you. If they aren't, there may be little reason to consider treatment outside of regular doctors' visits.

If your fibroids are presenting concerns, you have options. Some are less certain and may take a while to work, such as lifestyle choices and alternative medication; others have the benefit of treating your fibroids with relative speed, but require that you undergo a surgical procedure. Most drastically, you have a choice about whether to keep your uterus or not.

Many women, including myself, realize that they want to hold on to their uterus for either practical or emotional reasons, and often both. Of course, keeping your uterus means that you continue to have the option to become pregnant before menopause begins; but the uterus, as we saw on Day 2, also plays a structural role in your body, produces important hormones, and as we'll discuss more in Month 3, helps maintain sexual satisfaction.

Emotionally, some women identify strongly with their uterus; it represents a central aspect of their feelings of femininity and womanhood; it is an enormous component of sexual identity. Other women have a more dispassionate view of their uterus, and given the correct reasons, are able to envision and enjoy life without it.

No one approach is better or worse than any other, assuming you're making your decisions in conjunction with a trusted doctor. Many women simply don't realize they have a wide range of options with which they can manage their fibroids.

You can think of the range of fibroid treatments as a continuum, with "doing nothing" at one end of the spectrum and full hysterectomy at the other end, with six other points in between. You can combine some things, like lifestyle changes, with any of the other options.

THE TREATMENT CONTINUUM

□——□——□——□——□——□——□——□——□

Ignore It & Hope It Goes Away Watch & Wait Lifestyle Changes Alternative Treatments Drug Therapy Image-Guided Therapy Myomectomy Hysterectomy

You can choose whether to start at the beginning of the spectrum and move forward, step by step, or you may feel that you want to jump into a treatment option partway along the continuum. (The one thing I would not suggest, however, is starting at the far end, with **hysterectomy**, until you've at least explored or become fully informed about less drastic approaches to fibroid and symptom management. A hysterectomy is always an option, should you decide you want one. However, once you have a hysterectomy, you can't undo it.)

You also don't have to go step-by-step along the continuum. For instance, I started off with watchful waiting, moved into lifestyle changes, briefly explored **acupuncture** (an alternative treatment), and then jumped to **myomectomy**. In the five years between my fibroid diagnosis and surgery, I also lapsed from time to time back to the first point on the continuum: Ignore it and hope it goes away! But when symptoms or a sonogram brought me back to reality, I went back on track to a more active fibroid management program.

Whichever point you choose to enter the continuum, even if it's straight into surgery, it's important to know that you do have choices and those choices are largely up to you. Whatever you choose to do, of course, it should be in conjunction with a doctor you trust, and include talking over your choices thoroughly with your partner, family, or close friends.

Understanding your own feelings about your body and your lifestyle is one way to start evaluating where you want to start your fibroid management program. Some of the key questions you need to ask yourself include:

- Are my fibroids bothering me at all physically?
- Do I want to maintain the option of getting pregnant?
- Do I want to keep my uterus, even though I'm not interested in getting pregnant?
- Do I have the willpower to try slower therapies that can help my symptoms, like changing my diet or trying alternative medicine?
- Am I suffering enough from my fibroids that I want to deal with them right now?
- Can I deal with the idea of possibly having to treat new fibroids again in a few years?
- Is sexual satisfaction important to me?
- If I were to lose my uterus, would I want to keep my ovaries to avoid going on HRT?

○ Am I concerned about uterine or ovarian cancer in my future? Do I have strong reasons—like family history—to warrant my concern?

The answers to these questions can help you determine which types of treatment are most appropriate for your particular goals. Of course, these questions, and the suggested answers, are only guidelines . . . use them to develop your own approach to the treatment paths available. In the second part of this chapter, we'll take a brief look at all of the available options to give you an overview of what's available and how to start evaluating what's best for you. In other chapters, we'll go through each of the options in more detail.

If you said, *"Yes, my fibroids are bothering me physically,"* then you might want to consider:

○ Watch and wait
○ Lifestyle changes (alone or in combination with other therapies)
○ Alternative therapies (alone or in combination with lifestyle changes)
○ Drug therapy (alone or in combination with surgery)
○ Image-guided treatments, which shrink or kill off fibroids without physically removing them, including **Uterine Artery Embolization (UAE)** and **cryomyolysis**.
○ Myomectomy, which cuts out fibroids but keeps your uterus intact.
○ Hysterectomy, which removes your uterus and perhaps other parts of your reproductive system.

If you said, *"Yes, I want to maintain the option of getting pregnant,"* then you might want to consider:

○ Watch and wait
○ Lifestyle changes (alone or in combination with other therapies)
○ Alternative therapies (alone or in combination with lifestyle changes)
○ Drug therapy (alone or in combination with surgery)
○ Myomectomy

If you said, *"Yes, I want to keep my uterus, even though I'm not interested in getting pregnant,"* then you might want to consider:

○ Watch and wait
○ Lifestyle changes (alone or in combination with other therapies)
○ Alternative therapies (alone or in combination with lifestyle changes)
○ Drug therapy (alone or in combination with surgery)
○ Image-guided treatments*
○ Myomectomy

*Note: Some of these options, including UAE, may also preserve your option to get pregnant; while these treatments haven't been studied long enough to give a definitive answer, we'll look at the pros and cons in Month 9.

If you said, "Yes, I have the willpower to try slower therapies that can help my symptoms," then you might want to consider:

○ Lifestyle changes (alone or in combination with other therapies)
○ Alternative therapies

If you said, "Yes, I'm suffering enough from my fibroids that I want to deal with them now," then you might want to consider:

○ Image-guided treatments
○ Myomectomy
○ Hysterectomy

If you said, "Yes, I can deal with the idea of possibly having to treat new fibroids again in a few years," then you might want to consider:

○ Lifestyle changes (alone or in combination with other therapies)
○ Alternative therapies (alone or in combination with lifestyle changes)
○ Drug therapy (alone or in combination with surgery)
○ Image-guided treatments
○ Myomectomy

If you said, "Yes, sexual satisfaction is important," then you might want to consider:

- Watch and wait
- Lifestyle changes (alone or in combination with other therapies)
- Alternative therapies
- Image-guided treatments
- Myomectomy
- Supracervical hysterectomy, which removes just the top part of your uterus, leaving your cervix, ovaries, and Fallopian tubes

If you said, *"Yes, if I were to lose my uterus, I would want to keep my ovaries to avoid going on HRT,"* then you might want to consider:

- Supracervical hysterectomy
- Total hysterectomy, which removes your uterus, including the cervix, but leaves your ovaries and Fallopian tubes in place

If you said, *"Yes, I am concerned about uterine or ovarian cancer in my future,"* then you might want to consider:

- Radical hysterectomy, removing your uterus, along with the cervix, ovaries and Fallopian tubes

IN A SENTENCE:

> *Your choice of how to treat your fibroids—and yourself—is very individual; one size does not fit all.*

learning

An Overview of Your Treatment Options

AS WE'VE just seen, there are eight points on the treatment continuum, ranging from "Ignore it and hope it goes away," to "Hysterectomy."

Now that you've started thinking about which options on the treatment continuum may be right for you, let's take a short look at what each of these options actually entails. As you read about each of the items in this overview, you'll see where in the book to go for more in-depth information on the subjects that interest you most.

Your treatment options:

1. Ignore it and hope it goes away
2. Watch and wait
3. Lifestyle changes (alone or in combination with other therapies)
4. Alternative therapies
5. Drug therapy (alone or in combination with surgery)
6. Image-guided treatments, including Uterine Artery Embolization, myolysis, and cryomyolysis

7. Myomectomy, which cuts out fibroids but keeps your uterus intact. There are three different types of surgery you can have, depending on where your fibroids are located and/or their size:
   - **hysteroscopic resection**, which removes certain fibroids vaginally
   - **laparoscopic myomectomy**, which uses microsurgery
   - **abdominal myomectomy**
8. Hysterectomy, which removes your uterus, and perhaps other parts of your reproductive system. There are three "levels" of hysterectomy, which are:
   - **supracervical hysterectomy**, which removes just the top part of your uterus, leaving your cervix, ovaries, and Fallopian tubes
   - **total hysterectomy**, which removes your uterus, including the cervix, but leaves your ovaries and Fallopian tubes in place
   - **radical hysterectomy**, removing your uterus, with the cervix, ovaries, and Fallopian tubes

1. Ignore it and hope it goes away

Since you're already reading this book, I think it's safe to assume that you have already decided not to ignore your fibroids. While sometimes you may just want to forget about them—and you shouldn't think about them every minute—you already know that ignoring them is probably not the healthiest option.

2. Watch and Wait

This is a very acceptable option, especially if your fibroids are not causing any symptoms, or the symptoms are mild enough not to interfere with your lifestyle. The three crucial aspects of this strategy are:

1. Keeping a Lifestyle and Symptoms Indicator (see Day 3).
2. Keeping track of your menstrual periods and any fibroid-related symptoms in your Menstrual Period Diary (see Week 2).
3. Seeing your gynecologist anywhere from two to four times a year, and getting sonograms at least twice a year.

Your Lifestyle and Symptoms Indicator will help you track whether your symptoms stay the same, fluctuate, or get worse. Along with your Menstrual Period Diary, it will help you and your doctor evaluate such variables as pain, bleeding, unusual periods, and/or fatigue, in order to determine whether there are any connections between your lifestyle and your symptoms and which treatments, if any, may be appropriate.

If you really use your Lifestyle and Symptoms Indicator to keep a detailed record, you might be surprised at what you discover. I found that my own symptoms seemed to get worse during periods of serious stress and avoided treatment for a number of years by keeping track of how my symptoms fluctuated, getting worse and then better again when the stress subsided.

Having sonograms on a regular basis will add another measure of knowledge. As we discussed on Day 2, each sonogram can give you the measurement of your fibroids. Sonograms done on a regular basis (every two to six months, depending on your doctor's advice) can document any changes in your fibroids.

Make sure that you get a copy of your sonogram results from your radiologist or gynecologist, and file or clip the report to your Lifestyle and Symptoms Indicator. Standard sonograms give you results in two dimensions, and by using a ruler marked with centimeters you can draw a rough diagram. Draw each of the two dimensions with two lines; let the lines cross in the middle, so that you have a rough "x" or cross. Connect the four outside ends of the lines to form a circle or an oval.

Every three months, when I got a sonogram, I drew my diagram, showing just the largest fibroid, on the same piece of paper. The first time, the dimensions were the size of a small plum. Over the course of several years, it changed a little, but not much. When the little "plum" became an "orange," I started looking for treatment options; when the orange grew even bigger, I decided it was time to take action.

Not everyone's fibroids require any action, ever. I know one woman who's been "watching and waiting" for almost twenty years. You may find this strategy is your easiest option; on the other hand, some women may find that it creates anxiety and fear. If that's the case for you, make sure to check out Month 2, where we'll talk about some strategies to ease those anxious feelings.

3. Lifestyle changes (alone or in combination with other therapies)

Charting Your Fibroid Growth

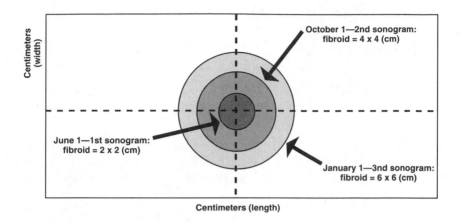

Over time, you can map the growth of your largest fibroid, using the dimensions provided by successive sonograms.

This strategy isn't any different from the ones you've read about in every magazine: diet, exercise, and stress reduction can all help make you healthier. But positive changes in each of these areas can also help your body fight fibroids more effectively, potentially helping to reduce symptoms and slow down fibroid growth.

Diet: As we saw on Day 5, certain foods can help your fibroids, while others can provide the fuel that helps fibroids grow. A healthy diet that stresses fruit, vegetables, and fiber is the core to your fibroid-fighting food plan; a complete shopping list for a fibroid fighting diet is shown in Day 5.

Exercise: As we discussed on Day 7, a regular exercise program can help you lose weight, control insulin, reduce cholesterol levels, and manage stress, all of which can help your body manage your fibroids more effectively. Write appointments for yourself in your calendar, at least three times a week, to walk, run, swim, dance, or whatever way you like to break a sweat.

Stress reduction: One of the least-talked-about side effects of fibroids is stress: anxiety, depression, fear, anger, and a host of other emotions. Managing stress can have an important impact on your attitude, which is an important part of your fibroid management technique; stress can also take a toll on your body in physical ways that can specifically affect your fibroids. We'll talk more about stress reduction techniques in Month 2.

4. Alternative therapies

Alternative therapies, including acupuncture, Chinese or Western herbalism, homeopathy, and Ayur-Veda, to name a few, seem to have more success treating fibroid symptoms than in reducing the size of fibroids or in making them go away. But for many women, symptom relief—whether of bleeding, pain, pressure, or stress—may be enough, and the gentler, slower aspects of alternative treatments may be soothing to the soul as well as the body.

We'll talk about many of the most popular alternative treatments for fibroids in Month 3.

5. Drug Therapy

There are three primary types of drug therapy available now, although several others are being tested. In addition, drugs being developed to target and kill cancerous tumors may someday be tested for their application to benign tumors, like fibroids. In the meantime, drug therapy consists of:

NSAIDS: primarily over-the-counter medications like aspirin, ibuprofen, and naproxen. These can help control mild symptoms, especially cramps and bleeding, by either slowing down the production of prostaglandins or by actually lowering estrogen levels. If you're experiencing very heavy bleeding or extremely painful cramps, you should see your doctor rather than self-medicating.

The Pill: low-estrogen birth control pills can sometimes help stop fibroids from growing; some doctors think the Pill can also be helpful in treating excessive bleeding or cramps. On the other hand, the Pill may make fibroids grow more. If you're on the Pill, or are considering it, talk to your doctor about the low-estrogen options, and monitor your fibroids on a regular basis.

GnRH Agonists: These are drugs which suppress all estrogen production in your body; essentially, they create a temporary menopause. Using a GnRH agonist can create a number of unpleasant side effects, but it does allow fibroids to shrink while you're taking the drug. When the treatment is stopped, estrogen returns, and fibroids begin to grow again. GnRH therapy can be effective if fibroids are preventing conception: the shrinkage can give prospective parents a window of opportunity to conceive without fibroids getting in the way.

Antiprogesterones: This is a class of drugs that suppress progesterone, the other major hormone besides estrogen that our ovaries produce, and one that recently has come under scrutiny for its role in fibroids' growth.

We'll discuss the various options in drug therapy—as well as some of the new developments currently on the horizon—in more detail in Month 4.

6. Image-Guided Treatments

There are a growing number of treatments which use a combination of pictures and probes to shrink or kill off fibroids without physically removing them. The "pictures" come from X-ray, ultrasound, or **magnetic resonance imaging (MRI)** machines, which allow doctors to get an image of your fibroids. The "probes" are inserted into a small incision in either your upper leg (for Uterine Artery Embolization) or abdomen; the doctor uses the probes to attack the fibroids. While these techniques are only mildly invasive, they can create some side effects.

Uterine Artery Embolization (UAE). In UAE, X-rays allow the doctor to guide the probe to the uterine artery. Tiny particles, each about the size of a grain of salt, are injected into the artery to cut down the blood supply to the fibroids, starving them of blood.

Myolysis and Cryomyolysis. These are two related techniques that, like UAE, kill off your fibroids while leaving them inside the uterus. Myolysis, also known as myoma coagulation, uses heat to kill the fibroid and its blood supply; cryomyolysis uses extreme cold. Myolysis and cryomyolysis are alternatives for women who aren't planning to have children in the future.

We'll review these procedures in more detail, especially UAE, in Month 9.

7. Myomectomy

You can think of myomectomy as a "fibroidectomy." Unlike the treatments covered in the previous section, a doctor performing a myomectomy removes fibroids from your uterus; unlike a hysterectomy, your uterus is kept intact or is repaired. Currently, myomectomy is the procedure most accepted for women who want to retain their option to get pregnant.

There are three variations on myomectomy:

Vaginal, also called **hysteroscopic resection**, is done if you have relatively small fibroids inside the cavity of your uterus. It's most effective for pedunculated fibroids, the kind that grow on a stalk from your uterine lining.

Laparoscopic uses microsurgery to identify and remove your fibroids. It is especially effective if your fibroids are inside the cavity or outside the uterus.

Abdominal is traditional, "open" surgery. It is especially effective for very large fibroids or fibroids in the wall of the uterus.

We'll review the different types of myomectomies, and the techniques available, in Month 10.

8. Hysterectomy

Doctors can perform hysterectomies just as they do myomectomies, either vaginally, laparoscopically, or using full abdominal surgery. The difference depends partly on the size and placement of your fibroids, and partly on your and your doctor's preferences. However, what all hysterectomies have in common is that they remove all or part of your uterus. Essentially, there are three types of hysterectomies:

○ **Supracervical hysterectomy**, which removes just the top part of your uterus. You keep your cervix, ovaries, and Fallopian tubes.

○ **Total hysterectomy**, which removes your uterus, including the cervix. You keep your ovaries and Fallopian tubes.

○ **Total abdominal hysterectomy**, which removes your uterus, including the cervix, ovaries, and Fallopian tubes.

We'll talk more about the details of hysterectomies—and the decision about whether to have one—in Month 11.

ON THE HORIZON

Several new therapies are in testing or have just been introduced for use. The long-term effects of these treatments are not known, but initial results indicate that they may become new options for fibroid treatment in the future.

Interferon. In a case reported in the medical journal *The Lancet*, a forty-two-year-old woman with chronic **hepatitis** was treated with a drug called interferon alpha; the woman also had a large fibroid, which was not treated separately. The woman received five months of interferon treatment for the hepatitis; by the end of that time, her large fibroid had shrunk to about 14 percent of its original size. The fibroid continued shrinking for another year, finally ending up at about 10 percent of its original size. There are side effects to interferon, which can include flu-like symptoms, weight loss, fatigue, and fever. The Center for Uterine Fibroids in Boston is planning further studies on the effectiveness of interferon as a treatment for fibroids.

A new drug called **Pirfenidone** may help block specific growth factors that can affect your fibroids. In early laboratory tests, it prevented the growth of fibroid cells; a study of the drug's effects on women with fibroids is currently being proposed to the FDA.

In March 2000, a new procedure called **I-MRI-guided cryosurgery** was first performed at the University of Mississippi Medical Center. This may represent an improvement on some of the image-guided techniques we discussed earlier. This procedure is performed with the help of a new type of MRI, which provides better visualization. While this procedure used extreme cold (cryotherapy) to kill fibroid cells, the important part may well be the use of improved imagery to target fibroids.

A similar test is being conducted using ultrasound instead of cryotherapy. Even more futuristic studies are being planned to see if fibroids can be treated with ultrasound from outside the body, without even breaking the skin.

Proton beam therapy is a treatment developed for cancer, but according to the editors of the *New England Journal of Medicine*, it "can be used for any solid tumor." It is a special form of radiation treatment which can target the unhealthy cells of a tumor, while largely leaving healthy tissue alone. Right now, proton beam therapy is available only at specific centers for cancer treatment.

IN A SENTENCE:

Your range of options for fibroid treatment exists on a spectrum; you can choose to go the full length of the spectrum, from the least invasive option to the most, or you can jump in wherever you decide is best for you.

Assemble Your Medical History

CREATING A medical history is an important and concrete step you can take to remain in charge of your medical care. In the beginning, everything is important, including as much as you're able to find out about the medical histories—such as any operations or illnesses—of your grandmother's, mother, aunts, and sisters. If possible, experts recommend going back as far as your great-grandparents.

In your own medical history, no detail is too small to leave out. This includes vitamins you take, herbs, homeopathic remedies, and as much of your past history as you can remember. You've already noted many of these items in your Lifestyle and Symptoms Indicator (Day 3); going forward, your Menstrual Period Diary (Week 2) will also be an important component of your medical history.

Your medical history gives you and your doctor a complete dossier on your health, including, to the extent possible, records of blood tests, sonograms, and other scans, and treatment by previous doctors. We'll look at how to assemble this information in more detail later in this chapter.

Whenever you see a doctor for the first time, you can take

your medical history along. You won't have to test your memory to remember the names of the medications you take, the milligrams in each prescription, or the dates of previous illnesses. The printed record will also give you a handy place to take notes of anything your doctor is saying. You'll feel confident and in control, which will influence the rest of your visit to the doctor.

If you create your medical history on your computer, you can easily make changes and print out new copies whenever necessary. Either way, keep one copy for yourself, and make a copy for your doctor.

Creating your medical history

1. Contact Information

At the top of the page, write down your name, age, address, contact information (phone numbers, e-mail address), and the date you last updated the record. Include your blood type, if you know it, allergies, and whether you use such items as contact lenses or hearing aids.

Examples

Birthdate:	*4/11/60*
Today's date:	*01/01/02*
Blood Type:	*0 neg*
Age:	*42*
Wear contact lenses/hearing aid/other	_____
Allergies:	*Hay fever*
	Penicillin

2. Current Symptoms

Recap symptoms from your Lifestyle and Symptoms Indicator; include such things as fatigue, weight loss/gain, and other side issues in addition to such items as bleeding, pain, and so on.

3. Medical History

This is your detailed record. The sample chart below shows a number of examples that will help guide you as you create your own history. For answers you don't know or don't remember, put a note such as "DK," for "don't know." This will remind you to research the answer later.

Sample Medical History

Medical Condition	When Diagnosed	Treatment, Including Medications and Dosage	Treating MD and/or Facility
CURRENT CONDITIONS			
Fibroids	3/01	n/a	Dr. Jane Doe phone/fax #s
High cholesterol	6/99	Lipitor 10 mgs	Dr Emily Smith phone/fax #s
Low thyroid	6/99	Synthroid, .1 mg	Dr Emily Smith
DES daughter	1970s	none	Dr John Black n/a
High blood pressure	Various	Taken off b/c pills	Dr. Jane Doe
OTHER COMPLAINTS			
Occasional headache	Aspirin	n/a	
Allergies		Antihistamine	
Other		Multivitamin	
Occasional stress		Bach flower remedy	
MEDICAL PROCEDURES			
Throat polyp	8/00	Outpatient surgery	Dr. An Yu phone/fax #s
Right Oopherectomy	6/76	Abdominal surgery	Boston Medical Center phone/fax #s
Birth control	[Date last fit]	diaphragm	

SUBSTANCE USE
(Note never/little/moderate/often); include past use and dates stopped

Alcohol _____

Tobacco _____

Illegal drugs _____

CHILDREN
(Note number, including none, if appropriate)

Dates born/ages _____

Medical conditions (if any) _____

Miscarriages (date/# weeks) _____

Abortions (date/s) _____

Charts/detailed reports: Attach copies of sonograms and other reports relating to your medical experiences.

Sample Medical History

Family history (include information for biologically related family members: it is not necessary to include in-laws, adoptees, spouses, or step-relatives)

Family Member	Known Conditions/ History (include operations, miscarriages, substance use, etc)	Cause of Death	Age at Death
Mother	Fibroids, high blood pressure	n/a (not applicable)	n/a
Father	High cholesterol	n/a	n/a
Sister(s)	none	n/a	n/a
Brother(s)	none	n/a	n/a
Aunt(s)			
Maternal	none	n/a	n/a
Paternal	n/a	n/a	n/a
Uncle(s)			
Maternal	n/a	n/a	n/a
Paternal	Diabetes	diabetes	67
Grandmothers			
Maternal	High blood pressure, stroke	Alzheimer's	83
Paternal	diabetes	car accident	68
Grandfathers			
Maternal	none	age	80
Paternal	tobacco	age	72
Great-grandparents			
Maternal	none known	stroke/age	dk
Paternal	none known	heart attack/age	98/45

Getting copies of your previous medical records, such as sonogram reports, liver tests, estrogen levels, and other blood work, may or may not be a challenge. The first step is simply to ask, preferably in writing, for copies of past medical records from your current and any previous doctors. Most hospitals and many doctors have a special release form that you can use to make your request. Be aware, however, that most states allow medical records to be discarded after a certain number of years; if you're looking for records from some time ago, call to find out if they are still available.

Some doctors keep meticulous charts on every patient; some are not as vigilant about writing everything down. Important items for monitoring your fibroids are:

○ records of medications prescribed.
○ records of sonogram, MRI, CT, or other imaging, including measurements of any masses found in your uterus or elsewhere.
○ results of blood tests, including **CBC** (complete blood counts, which show, among other things, whether you're anemic) and hormone profiles.
○ records of previous gynecologic surgeries.

Of course, you'll ask your doctor for all this information, but your best friend in getting these records may be your doctor's assistant or office manager. She'll have to ask the doctor's permission to release the information to you, but she is generally going to be more accessible than your doctor if you have questions or additional requests . . . and your doctor may be more likely to react quickly to her request than yours.

If you've been hospitalized in the past, you can also try calling the hospital for copies of your records. I was surprised when I was able, with one call, to get a copy of my records from the hospital where I'd had surgery over twenty years ago.

Be prepared if you encounter some resistance from your doctor. According to the website Cancerlinks, contrary to what you might naturally think, "medical records are the property of the health care facility, not the patient." Laws vary by state; some states require your health-care provider to furnish copies of your medical records on demand, but other states do not. In fact, "it can be surprisingly difficult to even get a good look at your medical records."

Here are some steps you can follow to make the process as straightforward as possible.

Call to find out to whom the request should be made. Whenever possible, it's best to get the name of an individual to whom you can write. You should also find out if there are any special things you need to do, such as have your letter notarized, or include a payment for postage or copying. Find out how long it usually takes to pull records, and how the records are sent. If records are usually sent out by regular mail, you can ask whether they can be sent by courier (such as Federal Express) or registered mail, or even if you can pick them up yourself. Get the name of the person who's giving you all this information so you can refer to her in your letter, and have a record of your conversation.

Send a letter. Make your letter brief and clear. It is helpful to include your full name (plus a notation if your name has changed), date of birth, Social Security Number, and date of treatment(s); you should also state that you are an adult over eighteen requesting your own records. Specify your request as precisely as possible, always asking for copies, not originals. (If originals are lost in the mail you have no recourse.) For instance, you may say, "I would like to receive copies of pelvic sonogram films made in April, 1998. My referring physician was Dr. A—, at (phone number) 212-000-1111." If the records are to be sent to a third party, such as another doctor, provide the name and address of that individual. Be sure to sign your request with your full name; include your phone number, billing address, and any other contact information, such as an e-mail address. If you prefer, you can write a letter for your current doctor to sign and send, requesting the records for her files.

If the doctor or hospital will not release your medical records, ask for a **written letter of denial**. Then contact a patients rights group, your state medical board, or an attorney for further assistance. At a minimum, the provider is usually required to send your records to a physician of your choice.

If you're still having problems, you can try sending a certified letter, requesting a copy of everything in your file. Mention the Federal Privacy Act, and note that you've sent copies to your state and local representatives.

Be cool. You already know it's true that you get more flies with honey than with vinegar. If you can, try not to let your fear, frustration, and possibly even anger get in the way of your goal: obtaining your records. If you encounter obstacles, be persistent but helpful. Try saying, "How can I help you make this happen?"

If you're really not getting anywhere, **ask one of your advocates** from your Fibroid Support Team to make a phone call or write a letter for you. My father once had a volunteer position doing exactly this; since he wasn't emotionally involved in the cases he was advocating, he was remarkably successful in getting things done for his "clients."

Keep a log. Make copies of all letters, e-mails, and back-up information that you send and receive; make notes of any phone conversations. Keep everything in a folder organized by date. This is the documentation you'll need to prove your claims in any arbitration.

Read the information you receive, and ask questions. Ask your doctor or an informed friend to review the material with you. If you see things you don't understand or that don't make sense, speak up. If you see mistakes or have questions that only the original provider can answer, make a copy of what you received. Mark it up clearly with your questions. Write an accompanying letter detailing the questionable information. Make another copy of both the marked-up records and your letter, and send it back to the office that provided it. Follow up by phone.

IN A SENTENCE:

> *Creating a complete medical history for yourself and your family can be a lot of work, but will put you in control of your medical records.*

learning

Check On Your Insurance Coverage

INSURANCE IN the United States is an issue with far more questions than answers. In the absence of universal—or even unified—coverage, how you handle your own insurance matters is going to be fairly individual, depending on your plan, your coverage, and even the state in which you live. But no matter what kind of health insurance coverage you have, now is the time to investigate what it will and won't potentially cover if you need medical treatment for your fibroids.

I made the mistake of assuming that the policy I had through my employer was comprehensive. I only found out a week before surgery was scheduled that I was mistaken, and I would be responsible for a bigger percentage of hospital charges than I had thought. So don't get caught in the same boat. Do your homework now, so you can either be assured that your policy will indeed cover all your medical expenses or you can investigate making some changes in your coverage. Either way, if you make a decision down the road that requires expensive treatment you'll know what you're up against.

Rhonda Orin, author of *Making Them Pay: How to Get the Most from Health Insurance and Managed Care*, also advises that you check the insurance laws in both your home state and the state in which you work. While state laws vary widely, and don't apply to people covered by federal health programs such as Medicare or self-funded plans run by employers, state laws do cover almost half of all insured families in the country. The laws can be hard to find, and to read. Ms. Orin suggests that if you're not comfortable with legal research, contact a consumer group in your area that works on health care issues (you'll find some national organizations listed in Month 12).

Doctor selection. The first question, of course, is which doctors you're eligible to see. A number of policies allow your ob/gyn to be your primary care provider. Depending on your policy, you may be limited to doctors who are on your plan, or you may be able to select your own doctor and receive partial reimbursement from your insurer. Before you have a big problem, take the time to find a doctor you like and trust. This requires time, money, and legwork, but if you're like me, you'll prefer having a qualified, compassionate doctor on board before trouble strikes.

If your plan requires doctor referrals, you should be able to ask your ob/gyn for recommendations and referrals to specialists in myomectomy, UAE, or other treatments. You can also ask to be referred to an **endocrinologist** for hormone evaluation and other specialists for blood count evaluation, imaging, and other tests.

Lifestyle management and alternative treatments. Find out if your plan covers alternative treatments such as nutrition or physiotherapy. My insurance plan allowed me to go to a chiropractor for relief of lower back pain brought on by my fibroids. Some plans may allow you to consult with a nutrition specialist to develop a healthier eating plan, an exercise physiologist to set up a customized workout schedule, a doctor qualified in Traditional Chinese Medicine, or a qualified specialist for acupuncture treatments.

"New" treatments. Insurance companies create their own definitions of what is "new" or "experimental" and therefore too risky, in their perception, to warrant coverage. This has been especially true most recently of Uterine Artery Embolization, and especially frustrating, because UAE has already been performed several thousand times in the United States, and is the subject of an increasing body of medical literature.

In March 2001, *The Oregonian* ran an article about a woman who was denied coverage for her UAE by a major carrier. She decided to fight the insurance company's ruling, appealing first to the insurance company, and when that didn't work, going to the state insurance commissioner's office, the governor's office, and patients' rights advocates. Six months after the initial denial of coverage, an independent panel ruled against the insurance company. While the ruling only covered this one case, the insurer later changed its policy for all women in the region.

The moral of the story: find out now which medical options your insurance carrier deems "appropriate," and if your treatment of choice isn't listed, start writing letters and calling both the management of your insurance company, and your elected officials, now. In addition to the information in this and other books, you can find articles in newspapers, magazines, or on the Internet that support your choice of treatment; make copies of these to include with your letters.

Hospitalization. Here's what I did wrong: I read my coverage and spoke to my insurance representatives by phone for pre-certification of surgery. I knew that since my doctor was "out of network" I would have to cover 20 percent of her charges. But since the hospital where she practiced was "in network," I believed that 100 percent of those charges would be covered. The insurance reps pointed out to me that my doctor's costs would only be partially covered. They never mentioned the hospital and—foolish me—I didn't think to ask.

A week before my treatment was scheduled, a patient care representative called me to make sure that all the pre-hospitalization steps were taken care of (we'll talk about these in more detail in Month 9). She confirmed that the doctor's cost was only partially covered. However, she informed me that the hospitalization was only partly covered as well. It turned out that the percentage of hospital costs covered flowed from the choice of doctor. The fact that the hospital was in the insurance carrier's network had no bearing.

Needless to say, I was not a happy camper. It was too late to do anything, since I did want the treatment, but I had to resign myself to a much higher bill than I'd originally anticipated.

So double-check everything in advance. If you are hospitalized, you can expect separate bills:

○ from the hospital, for room and board, and the services of the operating room;

○ from the anesthesiologist;

○ for lab work to analyze blood and tissue samples;

○ for any blood you may donate to yourself (I paid almost $100 a pint, an expense not covered by my insurance);

○ and of course, from your surgeon.

Find out in advance which of these services your insurance carrier will and will not cover, and at what rate (for instance, my out-of-network doctor—and subsequently, hospital—were covered at 80 percent of what is "reasonable and customary"). You should also find out how long a stay in the hospital is covered, and what the procedure is should you need to stay longer.

If you are not covered by insurance, either your own or a family member's, now would be a very good time to explore getting coverage that will, at a minimum, defray any surgical and hospitalization costs. You can often find group insurance programs through trade associations, religious groups, and other member-oriented organizations. (I found potential coverage through both the American Marketing Association and B'nai Brith.) To be eligible to join the insurance plan, which will require paying a premium each month, you will need to join the sponsoring organization, normally for only a few dollars per year.

IN A SENTENCE:

> *Find out about your insurance coverage before you need to use it for major procedures.*

FIRST-MONTH MILESTONE

By the end of your first month, you've begun sorting out specific treatment options, and laid the groundwork for any future medical treatments by:

- ○ UNDERSTANDING HOW YOUR LIFE GOALS CAN AFFECT YOUR CHOICE OF FIBROID TREATMENTS.

- ○ CREATING A MEDICAL HISTORY.

- ○ CHECKING YOUR INSURANCE COVERAGE.

Understanding the Mind-Body Connection

THERE'S ONE symptom of having fibroids that we haven't really covered in detail, and that is the emotions they generate: stress, anxiety, fear, self-recrimination, and other negative thoughts. Regardless of whether fibroids are creating physical symptoms, the emotional issues are ones almost every woman with fibroids has to deal with at one time or another. These are some of the fears I've had over time, and that other women have shared with me:

- ❍ fear of the unknown, that is, you didn't expect to get fibroids, and don't know what's going to happen next
- ❍ concern about your ability to get or stay pregnant
- ❍ fear of undergoing potential surgery or other treatments
- ❍ fear of losing your uterus
- ❍ fear of the impact on your relationships with partner, family, friends
- ❍ fear of losing or compromising your identity as a woman

In addition to these emotional reactions, having fibroids can cause stress in many other ways that affect your life:

O distraction from work or other responsibilities
O mental and/or physical exhaustion from worry
O moodiness or bad temper that affects the people around you
O stress-related behavior, like overeating
O physical symptoms that are the result of stress, such as insomnia

The effect of stress on your health may be affected by a combination of how strong the stressor is (a bad day at work versus a car accident, for example) and your personality. If you have a hard time expressing your feelings, or feel you have no one to talk to, or sometimes find it hard to stand up for yourself, stress may take a greater toll on your emotional health.

No surprise, women have high levels of stress. We're more likely to bring job stress home, and home is often a "second shift," with its regimen of cooking, cleaning, and chauffeuring. According to the *Mind-Body Health* newsletter, working women have an estimated twenty hours of work more per week than men have.

And how do we react to stress? Many women eat. One study found that "stressed emotional eaters ate more sweet, high-fat foods . . . than unstressed and nonemotional eaters." These food choices, over time, can, as we all know, compromise your health and provide more fuel for your fibroids.

So mind-body medicine can work at two levels:

O helping you deal with the emotional issues you are facing, which are very real, understandable, and treatable symptoms of having fibroids
O helping you understand and moderate your behavior to make sure you stay as healthy as possible

Can mind-body techniques cure your fibroids? I personally don't think they can cure you directly. I am also wary of mind-body techniques that blame you for your fibroids. Your fibroids are not your fault, and no amount of blocked creative energy or wounded child memories caused them to appear and grow.

Doctors exploring the use of mind-body medicine make a distinction between "curing" and healing." While mind-body medicine is unlikely to make your fibroids go away, that is, cure you, it may help you consider your life in new ways. Mind-body techniques can help you moderate certain physical habits, like how much (or little) you eat and sleep; you can also learn how to explore your thoughts and feelings more deeply. Indirectly, these techniques can lead you to better physical and mental health.

There is evidence suggesting that mind-body techniques help control or relieve stress, anxiety, and other emotions that can and do have an impact on our bodies. What's more, reducing stress can help you cope better with the demands of your daily life, and help you find new ways of taking care of yourself. Less stress can help you think with a clearer head about the true impact your fibroids are having on your life. You can be more effective at thinking through the kinds of treatments you think would suit you; you can be a better partner to your doctor, and help her be a better caregiver to you.

So where to begin? There are many constructive approaches, such as yoga, prayer, or massage, that can help you to de-stress. But even before starting on a specific program, let's look at six simple steps to help your mind start controlling your reaction to your fibroids . . . instead of your fibroids controlling your mind.

1. Take a time-out
2. Breathe
3. Think positively
4. Imagine what you want
5. Write it down
6. Reach out

Take a time-out

Many of us, when we have problems, prefer to stay busy, working even harder, cleaning even more, or whatever it is you do in order not to think about the thing that's bothering you most. It's not denial, exactly; it's more avoidance, a decision to put off a decision.

Bad news can also cause enormous anxiety, which in turn can lead to sleep problems, eating too much or too little, or taking out your fears and frustrations in inappropriate ways, like yelling at your partner or kids for no (especially) good reason.

The first thing I suggest doing when your mind starts racing, when your fears about fibroids are taking over your thoughts, when your anxiety starts affecting your behavior at work or at home, is just this: stop everything.

Your anxiety is like a speeding train; it's going so fast, and it's so single-minded, that it prevents you from being where you're supposed to be and doing what you'd normally be doing. So how do you get the train to stop?

Start with your body. Stop where you are, wherever you are, and close the door. Or go stand outside for a moment. Exhale. Exhale again, hard. Clear your mind. Gradually notice something about your surroundings, something small, some detail. What color the paint is. Where the chirping sounds of birds are coming from. Let yourself get re-anchored in the reality outside the whirling activity of your brain.

The time in my life when I was most beset by anxiety was not when I discovered I had fibroids (though that was high on the list); it was when I first separated, prior to going through a divorce. I still had to get up, get dressed, and go to work. But my enormous distress made it impossible for me to think about anything else. That's when I learned to stop.

I would sit at my desk and exhale. I would think about the one thing that I absolutely had to get done. And then I would do it. In the beginning, I had to take a short break between each task to get refocused. I had the freedom at work to leave and take a walk around the block or close my door for a few moments; that's a luxury, I know. But stopping to take a breath can be almost invisible to your colleagues. It can be relatively brief. You just have to make a conscious effort to stop that speeding train.

Eventually, the train will slow down on its own; eventually, you'll be in the engineer's seat, and manage the train yourself. But for now, just allow yourself a time-out.

Listening to music is one easy way to de-stress. In a study of patients undergoing eye surgery, listening to classical, folk, or even swing music brought their blood pressure down within five minutes.

There are other things you can do for yourself that can help you slow down, just a little. While you have more responsibilities than fingers and toes, you must add yourself to the long list of things and people you have to take care of. You must. Because just in case you think there's not enough time, or that you're not important enough, remember that you can't do anything for anybody else if you don't take care of yourself first.

So here are some suggestions for taking a short time-out. Which of these can you commit to doing once or twice this week? Which of your own suggestions would you add?

"Take a time-out" ideas
- ○ Close your eyes and take a deep breath. And another.
- ○ Take an hour off for lunch.
- ○ Take a drive.
- ○ Take a walk.
- ○ Stretch. Yawn. Sing.
- ○ Work in the garden.
- ○ Eat an apple (or a plum, or a pear . . .); do nothing else except sit and eat it.
- ○ Write a poem.
- ○ Go to a coffee bar; have a skim latte and read the paper.
- ○ Call a friend.
- ○ Turn off the ringer on the phone for half an hour.

You can think of other things, I'm sure. Whatever you choose to do, the idea is simple: take a look at how you spend the day, and figure out where you can grab five minutes for yourself—or more.

Breathe

Meditation is a longer, more focused version of taking a time-out. Meditation can take many forms: It can be a formal practice, as found in Eastern religions; it can take the form of prayer; it can be practiced using conscious, rhythmic breathing, chanting a personal mantra, or even by exercising.

According to Dr. Herbert Benson, President of Harvard's Mind-Body Institute and author of *The Relaxation Response*, "When a person engages in a repetitive prayer, word, sound, or phrase and when intrusive thoughts are passively disregarded . . . there is a decreased metabolism, heart rate, breathing rate, and slower brain waves." Studies have shown that meditation techniques can help relieve the effects of chronic pain, PMS, infertility, anxiety, and depression, among other things.

You don't need a guru to try meditation on your own. All you need is a quiet space. Sit peacefully and pay attention as you breathe in, then out.

Let any thoughts pass through your mind and return to your breathing. It can be helpful to find a phrase that you repeat. The classic Buddhist phrase is *om mani padme hum* (which means "the jewel in the lotus"), but you can pick a phrase from your own faith, a song, or a poem.

Meditation needs practice. Try it for a few minutes each day, just after you wake up, or just before you go to sleep. You can also meditate when you run, play the piano, or knit. Author Robert Ellwood cautions that meditation alone "will not magically remove the causes of anxiety, depression, or lethargy." But what it can do is help us stop the negative thoughts that slow us down, and rob us of energy and optimism. A daily ten-minute meditation may be as good for our minds as good food and exercise are for our bodies.

Think positively

A positive attitude is associated with a stronger immune system—and how well we take care of ourselves overall. In the University of Kentucky's famous Nun Study, nuns that expressed positive emotions lived as much as ten years longer than those who did not. David Snowden, director of the Nun Study, says "The more optimistic a person is, the less stress that person puts on his or her body over time."

Positive expectations can affect how well you weather a medical procedure. A study of women having **laparoscopy** (see Months 6 and 10), showed that the amount of pain they had could be predicted. The more each woman feared potential pain, the worse it seemed to be. A study of pregnant women found that those who felt able to handle the pain of childbirth may have had an easier time during labor and delivery.

Your doctor can also help influence your beliefs. In tests, people told by their doctors that a medicine would definitely work had much better results than patients whose doctors told them they weren't sure if the treatment would be effective. If your doctor says you *only* have an 80 percent chance of success, that may send a different message than saying, for instance, four out of five women have successful long term outcomes.

Imagine what you want

Shakti Gawain, in her book *Creative Visualization*, defines creative visualization as "using your imagination to create what you want in your life."

Why can this work? Because every action is preceded by a thought. You decided to learn more about fibroids, and then you spoke to your friends and started doing some research. You decided to buy a book, and you went to the bookstore, or jumped online, and did it.

Now, there is no evidence to suggest that visualization can shrink or remove your fibroids. On the other hand, do you want to see yourself eating more healthfully, exercising more, taking time out to relax? Visualization can help you "see" yourself there. Visualization can help put our minds on the positive track we'd like to be on—sooner or later, our actions follow. Visualization can also help relieve anxiety and reduce pain.

Hypnosis is a type of visualization in which you, or your therapist, clearly state your goals and focus on them over a period of time. You can go to a qualified hypnotherapist, but you can also try some self-hypnosis. A recent study suggests that self-hypnosis during childbirth may ease some of the pain of labor, lower the risk of medical complications, and reduce the need for surgery. The women in the hypnosis group said that practicing the technique gave them "a greater sense of control."

You can use hypnosis as a relaxation technique, a way to clear out everyday distractions and get in touch with your goals. You might want to start having a more positive attitude, put aside a past hurt, or envision a future success. It starts by getting into a receptive state. Then when you're ready, you tell yourself what to do; over time, you should see your suggestions taking hold.

Write it down

Novelist Cynthia Ozick has defined writing as "an act of courage." Keeping a journal means revealing your thoughts, feelings, and desires. It requires a certain amount of discipline. A journal is most effective when you write something every day.

Writing in a journal is a way of expressing yourself that's different from talking. You don't have to frame "perfect" sentences. You don't have to worry about how you sound or what you say. You have a rare opportunity to be completely honest, completely open, with no fear of recriminations or being misunderstood.

Writing is a powerful form of mind-body exercise. If you write about your fibroids without editing yourself, you may discover feelings you didn't even know you had: rage, anger, fear, guilt. Once you identify those feelings, you have a chance of dealing with them. Pouring your feelings out on a page (or on the computer) is a healthier response than repressing your feelings or acting on them inappropriately.

Another way to start putting your fibroids in perspective is to picture them—in color, with crayons and a big pad of paper. Sometimes pictures tap into elements of our subconscious that we can't articulate with words, even writing in a journal. During World War II, artist Charlotte Salomon told her life story in almost 800 small watercolor paintings; today, they are a masterpiece in which people can see both triumph and tragedy. When Charlotte entrusted the pictures to a friend for safekeeping, she asked him to guard them carefully. "They are my life," she said.

Your artwork doesn't have to be a masterpiece. But it can tell a story. So draw a picture of you and your fibroids (or make a collage, or a painting). After you make your drawing, step back from it and look at it objectively. What does it say about the person who made it? What would you counsel this woman to do if you thought she could use a new point of view? How would you like to change the picture?

Reach out

As we discussed on Day 4, reaching out to friends and community can also have a tremendous healing effect. In addition to friends and family, don't be afraid to contact a qualified therapist or nurse-practitioner to discuss your thoughts and fears about having fibroids.

Faith communities

People of faith, no matter which religion they practice, may have a powerful resource for creating a healthier body and spirit. Some faith traditions believe that faith alone can cure disease. Christian Scientists, for example, believe that God provides the "mental medicine" which heals the body; Pentecostalists rely on God as their primary "physician."

Other faith traditions don't promise physical healing, but offer a spiritual and emotional connection with both the divine and human forces around us. If you're part of a faith community, you can choose to ask members of your congregation to pray for you, cry with you, laugh with you—or just talk with you. People with a strong faith in God may have more hope, better coping skills, less depression—even enhanced immune function.

Faith can also play an important part in your medical care. A 1998 survey found that most people believe that prayer, meditation, or other spiritual practices can improve the results of medical treatment. At Duke University, doctors found that patients with some religious link had hospital stays that were only half as long as patients who didn't.

IN A SENTENCE:

> *Mind-body techniques can help you deal with your fibroids—and your life—in more creative ways.*

learning

Stress and Your Body

EMOTIONS CAN cause profound changes in both body and brain. Our bodies release hormones under stress that can suppress the immune system, impair memory, trigger skin problems, heighten muscle tension. When people are under stress, cuts and bruises tend to heal more slowly and latent viruses like herpes can become active again. Even thinking about stressful situations can cause stress hormones to rise; researchers in the United Kingdom found that the stress hormone **cortisol** was highest in their subjects on workday mornings. Cortisol helps the body respond to stress, but high cortisol levels can put wear and tear on the heart, brain, and other key organs.

Stress is also a key factor in infertility. Many of us know people who've struggled to get pregnant, only to have a biological baby after adopting. Or who have conceived while they were on vacation. Women dealing with infertility can have as much anxiety and depression as women dealing with heart disease, cancer, and HIV.

Can stress cause fibroids? Based on cancer research, it's possible that stress can be a factor in triggering disease in people who are already susceptible. So although it's probably not accurate to say that stress causes fibroids, if you're already predisposed because of your genes, body type, or other factors, stress might be the match that lights the fuse.

Can stress make fibroids grow? When animals were put in stressful situations—those in which they had no control or were helpless against repeated injuries—their tumors grew, an indication that feelings of having some control over our situations and having options are important for our health.

Improving your mood can affect your body as well. In an analysis of twenty-five years of data, doctors have shown that improving your mood can improve blood sugar control. There are two reasons for this. First, a better mood can mean that you're more likely to eat right, exercise, and focus on healthier habits overall. But secondly, it seems that depression can actually promote resistance to insulin, causing your body to produce increasing amounts. Apart from other health considerations, such as diabetes, extra insulin may help increase circulating estrogen, which can, as we've seen, affect your fibroids (see Day 5).

IN A SENTENCE:

> *Stress is not just psychological; It affects the body in profound physical ways.*

living

Can Fibroids Affect Your Sex Life?

THE UTERUS is a major part of our sexual system, and for many of us, a major part of our sexuality as well. When fibroids interrupt the natural workings, size, and shape of the uterus, they affect our sex lives very much indeed. Surprisingly, perhaps, this is not a subject that has been widely discussed until recently.

Often, we don't want to discuss something intimate, like problems in our sex lives, or something scary, like the possibility of having invasive surgery. When asked about their experiences in seeking help for sexual function problems, some 1,300 women gave overwhelmingly negative responses. One of the biggest issues for women dealing with reproductive tract conditions, such as fibroids, is our own reluctance to talk about our intimate concerns.

Doctors can also be at fault; many are uncomfortable discussing sex, and some are not willing to believe that fibroids can cause sexual problems. Laura Berman, assistant professor of urology and psychiatry at UCLA, tells us that "women reported that while doctors may listen to them, they don't feel like they were taken seriously."

Common wisdom, including among doctors, seems to be that the uterus has no part in sexual arousal, excitement, or satisfaction. Many doctors and even books will tell you that women's sexual response is largely a result of clitoral stimulation. Since this incorrect idea may affect your doctor's recommendation of treatments, it's important to know that the uterus is a key part of your sex life.

Sex and your uterus

When you start to get aroused, your heart beats faster and your adrenaline starts flowing. Your arteries dilate, filling your uterus, vagina, and the rest of your pelvic muscles with blood. The top third of your vagina swells while the uterus grows almost twice as big as it was before. And then your uterus actually starts to elevate, pulling up and back toward your spine; in the process, your vagina lengthens about an inch.

When you have an orgasm, the muscles of your uterus contract, clenching and unclenching in quick waves from the top of the uterus down to the cervix. Some women feel these contractions very strongly, defining the intensity of their orgasms by the strength of the contractions. The contractions, in turn, increase the pressure inside your uterus. The change in pressure alone can cause you to have another type of deeply felt orgasm. (You can experiment with creating and feeling sexual sensations in your uterus by stimulating your nipples or your G-spot [the coin-sized nerve center in the front wall of your vagina] which can cause uterine contractions.)

If you have multiple orgasms, one reason is that the blood flowing to your pelvis while you're still excited keeps your uterus enlarged and extended, which in turn keeps you primed for additional orgasms.

The cervix, the little ring of muscle that connects the neck of the uterus with the vagina, also plays a specific role in sexual pleasure for many women. One study found that almost half of the women surveyed were aware of orgasmic feelings from the cervix during penetration.

When the cervix is stimulated it contributes to sexual arousal and orgasm. Some of this is from the physical sensation that can occur during penetration; beyond that, this surprising little ring of tissue also releases **beta endorphins** during intercourse, heightening your feelings of pleasure and excitement.

The cervix also produces a thin mucus which provides about half the lubrication you feel during sex; fluid from your vaginal walls provides the rest. And if that weren't enough, scientists have identified a nerve, called the **vagus nerve**, which goes directly from the cervix to the brain stem. The vagus nerve is thought to be an independent pathway for the sensations of orgasm.

I've found that many women I've spoken with are not aware of the very important role the uterus plays in sex and orgasm. If you examine your own sexual responses, you may become aware of specific feelings of pleasure from your cervix and uterus.

How can fibroids affect your sex life?

Women have told me about a wide variety of problems that fibroids can cause during sex, including bloating, pressure, pain during penetration, a feeling that the uterus is shifting around, uterine, ovarian, and back pain. Fibroids can also affect your ability to have an orgasm, by preventing the uterus from being able to elevate, expand, or create contractions. On the flip side, one study did show—surprisingly—that women with nonsymptomatic fibroids were more sexually responsive, perhaps because fibroids increase the blood supply to the uterus.

Fibroids can make it hard for you to use birth control other than condoms and spermicide. If your fibroids have distorted the shape of your uterus, by tipping it back or changing the shape of the cervix, a diaphragm isn't an option, since it can't be fit properly and can also cause pain or pressure. As we'll see in Month 4, birth control pills may cause fibroids to grow.

Sometimes, fibroids can make even the idea of having sex less pleasant. The symptoms we discussed on Day 3, from bleeding to back pain, can affect any interest you may have in sex.

If you decide to treat your fibroids, what can you expect to happen to your sex life? In general, if you've been plagued by fibroid-related problems, your sex life should get better—simply because the pain or discomfort that prevented good sex has been relieved.

But how about your ability to achieve really great sex? Sad to say, in this sex-obsessed world of ours, women's sexual pleasure after fibroid treatment has only been studied in a limited way. There have been few if any studies conducted about sex before and after UAE, myolysis, cryomyolysis, or myomectomy. We know the most about sex after hysterectomy, but not how it compares to other, less invasive procedures. We'll go into the pros and cons of hysterectomy in detail in Month 11. But in the meantime, keep in mind that sex is a whole-body experience, including your uterus.

IN A SENTENCE:

> *The uterus is an important part of your sexual experience; fibroids can affect the quality of your sex life.*

learning

Fibroids and Alternative Medicine

IF YOU'RE like many women, the idea of trying alternative remedies to treat your fibroids may be very appealing. Therapies such as massage and acupuncture often take place in soothing environments, sometimes even by candlelight, or with soft music playing. Unlike our perceptions of Western medicine, alternative therapies can seem seductively "natural." (Although keep in mind that natural does not always equal "safe," or even "better"; as we'll see, it's important to do your homework and work with qualified practitioners.)

Alternative remedies tend to be more effective at relieving fibroid symptoms than in making fibroids go away. If your fibroids are small and your symptoms moderate, alternative

---

ALTERNATIVE MEDICINE is a catch-all phrase for a huge variety of treatments from a wide range of traditions, none of which are considered standard in Western medicine. Some of these treatments include acupuncture, massage therapy, biofeedback, megavitamins, homeopathy, spiritual healing, folk remedies, and "energy" healing using touch, magnets, or other devices.

remedies can offer relief for bleeding, cramps, and fatigue. It's important to tell your doctor what you're doing, whether you're trying acupuncture, herbal medicine, or some other therapy. She may have input for you from medical literature or her experience with other patients; you may also be able to add to her store of knowledge.

Many women manage their fibroids quite comfortably for years, using a combination of lifestyle improvements (such as we discussed on Days 5 and 7) and some of the alternative treatments we'll look into in this chapter. You should continue to go to your gynecologist for check-ups on a regular basis and ask for an ultrasound every three to six months to monitor fibroid growth.

If your fibroids are quite large, or your symptoms severe, you may want to try alternative therapies, but you should monitor your symptoms very carefully, using the Lifestyle and Symptoms Indicator, as well as your Menstrual Diary, we discussed on Day 3 and Week 2. Stay in close communication with your doctor and become well-informed about the medical options available (see Months 9, 10, and 11), in case you and your doctor decide it's time to try more aggressive treatments for your fibroids.

Alternative remedies are not magical. Unlike Western medicine, alternative remedies are not regulated, nor are there many "proven" results, such as those offered by the traditional peer-reviewed studies done by medical doctors in controlled tests. Since so little is known about most alternative therapies, it's wise to find out all you can about the therapy you'd like to pursue, and the practitioner you plan to work with—just as you would with any type of medical procedure and surgeon.

Both Western medicine and alternative remedies have a lot to offer— and a lot to be cautious of. What's interesting is how much the two approaches can potentially complement each other in your total health care. One sensible approach is to explore alternative therapies with a qualified practitioner without neglecting what Western medicine has to offer.

There are many alternative practices that promise relief for fibroids or fibroid symptoms, but few show any documented evidence of success. Some of the most popular alternative remedies, however, do offer enough information to let us look at the pros and cons of each. Many of these therapies, as we'll see, are based on similar philosophies, and include sound suggestions for living healthier lifestyles. Remember though, that these "alternative" remedies are not "do-it-yourself." Before starting any

What is attractive about alternative therapy for fibroids?
- Evaluates and treats your fibroids as part of a larger system
- Works on the theory of **homeostasis**—that the body needs to be in balance for proper functioning
- Herbs, homeopathic, and naturopathic remedies are often tailored specifically to you
- Usually involves a calm, relaxing treatment environment
- Treatment does not usually include serious side effects during or after the procedure
- May work best on symptoms like bleeding and cramps
- Seems to work best on smaller fibroids

What should you take into account?
- Generally takes some time to work
- Needs to be part of an ongoing routine; stops working when you stop treatment
- Virtually no comparative studies or large-scale trials
- No proven track record for results treating fibroids
- There is no pharmaceutical regulation for herbs or creams; potency can vary widely
- Most treatments are not covered by insurance

treatment, please consult a qualified practitioner (you'll find resources listed in Month 12).

- Western Herbalism
- Traditional Chinese Medicine (TCM), including Chinese herbalism and acupuncture
- Homeopathy
- Naturopathy
- Ayur-Veda

Western herbalism

Plants heal. We rely on the natural world to treat everything from breast cancer to mosquito bites. Up to 30 percent of the medications that doctors prescribe every day come from plants; Americans spend over $4 billion a year on vitamins, supplements, and herbs to heal or prevent illness, and many of us find relief. In my own medicine cabinet, I have aloe and tea tree oil for burns and scrapes; witch hazel for mosquito bites; and gelcaps of garlic, flaxseed, and omega-three oils.

Over the protests of the FDA, Congress exempted herbal products from FDA regulation in 1994; as a result, there are wide variations in preparation, potency, dosage, and delivery form (for example, pill versus capsule), all of which affect how well these herbs work. A recent study found herbal remedies in stores contaminated by bacteria or fungi; these could pose health risks, especially if your immune system is compromised. (FYI, the most contaminated source of herbs in the study were the open bins in a natural foods store.)

As herbal remedies become more popular, some natural sources are becoming scarcer and more expensive. In order to keep costs down, some manufacturers dilute the potency of the herb with other substances; chemical tests have shown that some brands use none of the herb listed on the label. Some products are mixed with medicines such as steroids, sedatives, and hormones . . . without revealing the presence of those ingredients. Thus, it's entirely possible, according to Jane Brody, writing in *The New York Times*, that "countless consumers are wasting their money on useless products or jeopardizing their health on hazardous ones."

Last but not least, herbs that are prepared and packaged properly are still medicinal substances. Though usually not as strong as prescription medicines, many plants have naturally-occurring chemicals that can be habit-forming, harmful, or cause individual allergic reactions.

For all of these reasons, I recommend consulting with a qualified practitioner before starting a regimen of herbal medicine; you should also tell your doctor about any herbs you plan to take. You may also want to pick up a good herbal reference book, such as *Tyler's Herbs of Choice*, by James E. Robbers and Dr. Varro E. Tyler, or the *Physicians' Desk Reference for Herbal Medicines*, which draws on German research to document the facts behind more than 600 botanicals. Other resources are listed in Month 12.

If your fibroids are causing problems, and you haven't yet reached menopause, herbal remedies may help you reduce bleeding, ease cramps, cleanse your system, and perhaps even shrink your fibroids. Often, a practitioner in herbal medicine will recommend a mixture of several herbs to accomplish your goals, taken according to a specific schedule. You'll need some patience to see if your herbal remedy is working; it can take weeks or months to show effects.

Some cautions:

○ If you've already reached menopause, herbs and other sources of phytoestrogens taken in large amounts may make your fibroids grow or cause bleeding. If you're on HRT, GnRH agonists, or birth control pills, phytoestrogens can block the effects of those drugs.

○ Herbs can interact with prescription or over-the-counter medicines just like "regular" medicine; this can potentially lead to dangerous drug interactions or overdoses.

○ A number of herbs can cause bad reactions, especially if you're pregnant or have a systemic disease like lupus or HIV.

○ Some plants have an effect like estrogen; others mimic progesterone. Depending on your own levels of these hormones (which vary over time), these herbs may cause an imbalance in your levels of estrogen and progesterone. Remember, as we discussed in Week 2, that fibroids may get bigger and bleed more as a result of imbalanced estrogen or progesterone, so be prepared to watch your symptoms carefully.

Herbs that may help

The following list shows a number of different herbs and the symptoms they may help relieve. Herbs come in different strengths and formats, including raw or dried plants, liquids, capsules, powders, and teas. If you're using the natural plant to make tea, Laurel Vukovic, author of *14-Day Herbal Cleansing*, offers the following tip: most roots and barks should be simmered in boiling water, covered, for 15–20 minutes, while leaves, flowers, or seeds should be put in the bottom of a teapot, covered with boiling water, and left to steep for fifteen minutes or so. Keeping the pot or teapot covered is important, so that healing properties aren't lost with escaping steam.

Herbs that may shrink fibroids:
○ Echinacea

O Garlic
O Sequoia buds
O White ash
O Yarrow

Herbs that may control cramps:
O Black haw
O Cramp bark
O Garlic
O Ginger
O Hops
O Partridgeberry
O Raspberry leaves
O Skullcap
O Valerian
O Yarrow

Herbs that may control bleeding:
O Beth root
O Cinnamon
O Cramp bark
O False unicorn root
O Lady's mantle
O Nettle
O Partridgeberry
O Shepherd's purse
O Yarrow

Herbs to use cautiously, or not at all

The herbs in the following list are popular traditional remedies for fibroids, bleeding, or cramps, that simply may not be good for your fibroids, or could have risky side effects. Scientists have found that three popular herbal therapies—black cohosh, chaste tree (vitex), and dong quai—can increase the size of the uterus or make uterine cells divide. Since a fibroid starts from just a single uterine cell, helping those cells grow or divide is not something you want to do.

More extensive studies of these herbs are underway. In the meantime, here is what we know about these popular remedies, and how they can affect your fibroids.

○ **Black cohosh** is used in a popular form of HRT known as RemiFemin®, as well as other brand name preparations. In the United States and Germany, black cohosh is the herb that is prescribed the most for treating symptoms of menopause. Some studies say that black cohosh does not "replace" estrogen; it may in fact work on the brain, affecting the hypothalamus, the brain's regulator of estrogen and body temperature. Most telling for women with fibroids, the research from the University of Pittsburgh has shown black cohosh can make uterine cells divide, as well as make bleeding and cramps worse.

○ **Chaste tree**, or vitex agnus-castus, is often recommended for regulating heavy bleeding and shrinking fibroids; it's also said to be calming and relaxing. Like black cohosh, chaste tree can cause uterine cells to divide. Chaste tree may also increase progesterone levels, which as we saw in Week 2, may make fibroids grow faster. In addition, if you're taking birth control pills, chaste tree may make them ineffective.

○ **Dang gui** (also called angelica or dong quai) has gained popularity as an almost all-purpose "woman's remedy." Its benefits include regulating menstruation and relieving cramps, stabilizing blood sugar levels, and enhancing the function of the immune system. However, according to Dr. Susan Love, you should avoid dang gui if you have heavy menstrual bleeding, or fibroids.

If you have high blood pressure, cardio-vascular problems of any kind, or heavy bleeding, be very cautious about using the following:

○ **Blue cohosh** is a traditional Native North American remedy for cramps. In research, blue cohosh did not promote uterine growth, but it was shown to raise blood pressure and constrict the blood vessels leading to the heart.

○ **Licorice** (the herb, not the candy) is a well-known phytoestrogen that in tests did not promote uterine growth. However, it can raise your blood pressure, more so if you're on the Pill, and can only be safely used for 4–6 weeks, or under a doctor's supervision.

○ **Motherwort**, recommended by some sources as a beneficial uterine tonic, may make bleeding worse.

Traditional Chinese Medicine (TCM)

Traditional Chinese Medicine (TCM) has been practiced for over 2,000 years (you may also hear of a simplified version of TCM, developed in Japan by Buddhist monks, called Kampo). TCM is based on the concept of balancing **Qi** (pronounced "chee"), the life force that flows both around and through us. Qi is made up of two equal but opposite forces called yin and yang; these need to be in balance for perfect health. Yang is the half of Qi associated with heat, dryness, light, action, and expansion. Yin is cold, damp, dark, and quiet; it's associated with the earth, interior, and deficiency. The liver, which in TCM is said to regulate fibroids, is a "yin" organ. (The liver also plays an important biological role in controlling fibroid growth by filtering excess estrogen out of our systems.)

According to TCM, fibroids are the result of blocked energy in the liver and gall bladder, the organs that are in charge of regulating all growth, both wanted and unwanted. When growth of any kind—including spiritual and emotional growth—is unbalanced, either by being repressed or out of control, the energy of the liver becomes blocked. In response, the liver creates an "overgrowth" somewhere in the body, such as fibroids. (Since Qi is responsible for moving the blood, this block is also called Blood Stasis, or blood stagnation.)

A TCM practitioner will work with you to balance your yin and yang, creating a state of physical and mental balance known as homeostasis. A skilled TCM practitioner will look for a Pattern of Disharmony, by taking your pulse, observing your face, tongue, and body, evaluating how you describe yourself and your symptoms, and asking you specific questions about your physical, mental, and emotional health.

Depending on your own Pattern of Disharmony, treating your fibroids might require clearing away accumulated heat (yang), or reducing too much cold (yin), thereby allowing the Qi to flow freely. If your fibroids are very small, TCM might be able to make them go away, but in general, TCM seems to be most helpful for treating symptoms, regardless of the size of your fibroids. TCM practitioners look at healing as a process; treatment for fibroids can range anywhere from six to eighteen months.

The most common treatment methods in TCM are acupuncture and Chinese herbalism; your practitioner might recommend one or both of these methods to treat your fibroids or fibroid symptoms.

Acupuncture. This method is most consistently successful in treating pain or bleeding from fibroids, although it is sometimes used to slow the growth of smaller fibroids. The World Health Organization endorses acupuncture to treat frequent or heavy bleeding, and the NIH (National Institutes of Health) has found that acupuncture may release natural pain killers (endorphins) and is helpful for a number of conditions, including low-back pain and menstrual cramps, although since the process takes time to work, you might not get relief from these symptoms for up to six months.

Acupuncture doesn't hurt, though you might feel pin pricks when the needles go in. Some therapists apply a low electric current to the needles to stimulate the acupoints even more; I've also found this to be painless.

Your therapist may combine acupuncture with other techniques to strengthen the healing process, such as pressure (**acupressure**), burning herbs (**moxabustion**), or Chinese herbs, taken as pills or teas.

It's important to make sure you work with a licensed acupuncturist. In addition, both Western physicians and traditional acupuncturists caution that you should consult—or at least inform—your primary physician about all treatments.

Chinese herbalism is also practiced according to the balancing principles of yin and yang; again, the secret is determining and treating the cause of disharmony. Age and your own personal body chemistry are very important factors in Chinese herbalism, as they are in Western herbalism. For instance, remedies used for menopausal symptoms may not be appropriate for women who are still menstruating.

Much of what is reported about the success of Chinese herbal medicine for fibroids is based on a handful of studies done in China and Japan. While not definitive, the results are encouraging:

○ In one study among 100 women, a traditional Chinese remedy called Kuei-chih-fu-ling-wan (also Keisha-bukuryo-gan in Japanese, or KBG) improved bleeding 90 percent of the time and shrank fibroids 60 percent of the time.

○ ∕ In another study using KBG and a Kampo formula called Shakuyaku-kanzo-to, bleeding problems were "moderately improved" in 60 percent of women with moderate to small fibroids. The treatment did not work on women with larger fibroids. (Shakuyaku-kanzo-to alone is said to be effective for menstrual pain and cramps; since it contains licorice, it should not be used by women with high blood pressure.)

○ Another study of 223 women with fibroids reported that individualized herbal treatments reduced heavy menstrual bleeding for at least half the women who had this problem, reduced the size of fibroids significantly for about a third of the women, and actually helped fibroids disappear for a small group. Overall, the treatment helped over 85 percent of the women in the study.

○ A remedy called Xiaoliu Tablet (XLT) was studied by doctors affiliated with Shanghai University. In a study of 71 women with fibroids, the study claimed "good results" in reducing the size of fibroids, especially if they were small.

In addition to individualized herbal preparations, there are a number of standardized formulas (see box) for fibroid treatments. A wide variety of natural, if not always appetizing, ingredients may be found in these formulas: One recipe for a tea, to be taken once a day for ninety days, calls for various amounts of peony root, Chinese angelica, myrrh, peach kernels, safflower—plus several grams each of leeches and flying squirrel feces.

You may be asked to avoid certain foods while you're taking your herbs: for instance, while taking the combination of herbs and other natural substances called Xiaoliu Tang, you are advised not to eat "seafood or any other fishy, dry, hot, or pungent food." While taking Fu An Tang, you are advised not to eat leeks.

It's important to consult a qualified herbalist or TCM practitioner before starting treatment. If you're pregnant, you should be extremely cautious about taking Chinese herbs. Of course, if you're taking any medications or have any health conditions, consult with your doctor about any possible interactions.

Homeopathy

Homeopathy is an alternative healing method that actually defies Western medical thought. According to the *New England Journal of Medicine*,

Standardized TCM and Kampo Remedies

MANY OF these treatments are commercial preparations said to help treat fibroids or their symptoms. They may be prepared as teas, capsules, or powders to mix with water. Ask your TCM practitioner about efficacy, possible side effects or allergic reactions, and doses before trying on your own.

TO CONTROL FIBROID GROWTH

- Xiaoliu Pian
- Xiaoliu Tang (Tumour Removing Decoction)
- Cinnamon and Persica C. (Uterine Myoma Formula)
- Reishi medicinal mushroom formula
- Keisha-bukuryo-gan, also known as KBG, or Kuei-chih-fu-ling-wan
- Shao Fu Zhu Yu Tang (Cinnamon and Bulrush C.)

TO CONTROL BLEEDING

- Shen-qian gu-jing granules
- Yun Nan Bai Yao
- Keisha-bukuryo-gan, also known as KBG, or Kuei-chih-fu-ling-wan
- Shao Fu Zhu Yu Tang (Cinnamon and Bulrush C.)

TO PREVENT CRAMPS

- Gui Zhi Fu Ling Wan (Cinnamon and Hoelen F.)
- Shakuyaku-kanzo-to

GENERAL FIBROID TREATMENTS

- Fu An Tang (Woman's Safety Decoction)
- Bai Xiao Dan
- Xue Jie Capsule (Dragon's Blood Capsule)
- Blue Citrus
- Chih-ko and Curcuma C.

there is not only no objective proof that homeopathy is effective, but it is based on principles that "violate fundamental scientific laws."

Homeopathy tells us that the body is integrated by a "vital force" which maintains a state of health. Illness is not considered unhealthy, but a sign of the body restoring itself to balance. Homeopathic therapy is intended to stimulate the self-healing process.

Homeopaths divide us into at least fifteen different types of personalities, based on looks, temperament, even body temperature; different types of people tend to get different homeopathic remedies.

Remedies are chosen according to the "law of similars." After diagnosing an illness, a homeopathic practitioner will create a remedy made from ingredients which, in their original form, would induce symptoms similar to those of the illness. However, in a twist that some people find baffling, homeopaths *dilute* these ingredients to increase their potency: some remedies might contain nothing of the original substance. This dilution is the reason many Western doctors question whether homeopathy can have any real medical effect.

As to whether homeopathy can treat fibroids, the *Consumer's Guide to Homeopathy* says that "homeopathic remedies for fibroids will not always completely get rid of them, but they do often reduce bleeding or other complications. Homeopathic treatment of fibroids tends to be more effective when [the fibroids] are not too extensive."

If you're interested in trying homeopathy to treat your fibroids, once again, it's important to find an experienced practitioner. If you're taking any prescription medicines, don't start homeopathy before talking with your doctor; if you're on birth control pills, you may not be able to use homeopathy effectively.

One aspect of homeopathy you can explore on your own, if you choose to, is diet. Homeopathic practitioners believe that fibroids, as well as other growths in the body, correspond to an overly acidic body chemistry; a homeopathic diet can help bring your system back into balance. As it happens, the foods that can make your body too acidic include many of the same foods that, as we saw on Day 5, should be consumed less often by women who have fibroids, including coffee, alcohol, meat, dairy, and sugar.

A basic homeopathic diet includes many of the same "good" foods we discussed on Day 5: whole grains, beans, cooked vegetables, and perhaps some low-fat animal protein, depending on your homeopathic body type.

Naturopathy

Like homeopathy, naturopathy is based on the principle that our bodies have the power to heal themselves. Naturopaths also believe our bodies have a natural equilibrium, or **homeostasis**, that can be upset by an unhealthy lifestyle.

Many naturopathic ideas have been so incorporated into our way of thinking that they now seem like common sense. For instance, naturopaths suggest that an unhealthy diet, lack of sleep, exercise, or fresh air, emotional or physical stress, pollution, and even negative attitudes can allow waste products and toxins to build up in the body, upsetting homeostasis, and creating illness.

For fibroids, a naturopath may suggest a diet low in fat and high in fiber to encourage elimination of excess estrogen; if you're bleeding heavily, you might also be advised to eat iron-rich foods to prevent anemia. You may also be prescribed herbal remedies, yoga, massage, and sitz baths.

Ayur-Veda

The healing system known as Ayur-Veda is thought to have originated 5,000 years ago: some call it the "mother of all healing" for its influence on Chinese, Greek, Western, and holistic medical theory.

Ayur-Veda divides us into three primary types based on both physical and emotional characteristics. These three types are called Pitta, Vata, and Kapha. Kapha-type women are thought to be the most likely to get fibroids; they may be advised to modify their diets by eliminating dairy and reducing red meat, salt, caffeine, alcohol, and heavy foods.

Regardless of your body type, fibroids are thought to be the result of poor digestion; in Ayurvedic terms, digestion is a complicated process involving the mind as well as the body. In Ayurvedic medicine, a healthy digestion influences **ojas** (also called **prana**), which is the rough equivalent of Qi, the life force that keeps our bodies in balance.

Improving your digestion requires adjusting both your mind and body. Depending on an analysis of your condition, an Ayurvedic practitioner may recommend a detoxifying program that could include laxatives or enemas, Ayurvedic herbal remedies, and restorative techniques such as therapeutic massage, yoga, meditation, and sunbathing.

Tapping into your chakras

The chakras are an energy system that, like Ayur-Veda, were defined by Hindu philosophers in India thousands of years ago. Seven chakras ascend from your groin to the crown of your head; each one is linked to specific parts of the body and different emotions, colors, and earth elements. Yoga was designed to release and stimulate **kundalini**, the energy that unblocks and balances the chakras.

The second chakra, called the Sacral, or Hara, is the one most related to the uterus. Located in the lower abdomen, about three finger-widths below the navel, the Sacral chakra energizes a range of sensual forces—our creativity, our sexuality, our ability to be playful, our capacity for joy. Blocked or imbalanced energy in the second chakra can result in fibroids. Jim Gilkeson, author of *Energy Healing: A Pathway to Inner Growth*, writes that the second chakra "relates to emotional control." When the chakra is functioning properly, we are calm, but if the chakra is in poor condition, we are more likely to become enraged and "out of control."

The color of the second chakra is orange. A meditation where you imagine breathing in bright orange light can help balance this chakra; orange foods and liquids are also thought to be strengthening. Water is also strengthening: you can drink a glass of water slowly, take a warm bath, or if possible, look out onto a river, sea, lake, or brook for a few minutes of calming reflection.

There are several yoga postures associated with the second chakra, including the Pelvic Lift, Triangle, or Moon; these poses encourage circulation in the pelvic region and may help ease symptoms like bloating or fullness.

You can also try cleaning your chakras. I found relief from mild cramps using this exercise, adapted from *Shaman, Healer, Sage*, by Dr. Alberto Villoldo:

While you are in a warm shower, hold your hand several inches above your skin, palm toward your body, two to four inches below your belly button. You may feel a dense knot of energy: this is your Sacral chakra. Move your palm in a slow circle, going counter-clockwise; feel yourself cleaning the accumulated dirt on your chakra. When you're ready, hold up your hand to the shower, so that the running water can clean off the toxic energies.

Next, put your hand back in the same position over your belly, but this time move it in a clockwise direction three or four times, to make the chakra spin properly.

When you're done, say "Aaahhh"; that is the relaxed, happy sound associated with a clean Sacral chakra.

IN A SENTENCE:

> There are many alternative remedies for fibroids and their symptoms that you can try before moving on to stronger medical treatments.

Considering Drug Therapies

DRUGS PRESENT a particular dilemma for women with fibroids. Stronger than herbs, certain drugs replace or control our natural hormones in order to help reduce fibroid symptoms, temporarily shrink the fibroids themselves, or if you decide to have a hysterectomy, replace some of your natural hormones. However, most drugs do include the risk of side effects, and virtually all must be taken continually in order to be effective.

As we saw in Week 2, your own hormone levels may be higher or lower than "average," yet still be perfectly normal for you. This variation may play a big role in determining how certain drugs, such as the birth control pill, may affect your fibroids.

In addition, different types of drugs can be more helpful at one time of your life versus another. If you decide to explore drug therapy, your age and life goals will play a part in your decision of what to take, and how it will affect you. Remember, there are no panaceas and you must work carefully with your doctor to make sure each of your choices along the way are the right ones for you.

In this section, we'll explore the various choices available and appropriate for women at different life stages; later, in the

Learning section, we'll review all of the benefits and drawbacks of each drug in more detail.

Teen to mid-adult years

From your teens through your middle adult years, if you're like most women, your ovaries are producing normal amounts of estrogen, progesterone, and other natural hormones. If you develop fibroids during these years, regulating or changing the amount of hormones your body produces may help reduce your symptoms, and possibly even keep your fibroids from growing.

The birth control pill is often recommended by doctors in these years, especially to help control heavy bleeding or reduce cramping. The birth control pill replaces the natural hormones in your body with low doses of artificial estrogen and progesterone; since you take the same amount each day, it also evens out the natural fluctuations in your hormone levels, that as we discussed in Week 2 can cause your fibroids to grow.

Studies on how the birth control pill affects fibroids are mixed; some suggest that they can make fibroids grow, while others show that fibroids and symptoms such as heavy bleeding are controlled. As with other types of drug therapy, it's important to monitor your fibroids' growth, if any, through regular sonograms.

Of course, these are also the years when women who want biological children will try to get pregnant. If you have fibroids, sometimes drugs called GnRH agonists are used to shrink fibroids temporarily, giving you a window to get pregnant right after the treatment is stopped. The same result, possibly with fewer side effects, can be achieved with a drug called mifepristone, more popularly known as RU-486. We'll be reviewing these treatments later in this chapter.

Perimenopause

This is a term used to describe the stage of life beginning anywhere from five to ten years before menopause. Every woman's timing is different, but most women begin to go into perimenopause between their late thirties and late forties. As we discussed in Week 2, this is the time when your estrogen and progesterone may be most out of balance and your fibroids are most likely to go through growth spurts.

Taking birth control pills at this stage of life can help even out these hormone fluctuations, helping to prevent rapid fibroid growth and increased symptoms.

If you and your doctor think that you're close to menopause, GnRH agonists can temporarily shrink your fibroids by cutting down your body's production of hormones before your body takes over doing that naturally.

GnRH agonists are also used to shrink fibroids before fertility treatments.

Postmenopause

This is the term used for when your hormones have declined to their lowest levels, although your ovaries continue to produce small amounts of hormones. Fibroids usually shrink at menopause, due to the lower levels of estrogen and progesterone in your body, and symptoms may disappear, but the fibroids themselves don't necessarily go away.

When you reach menopause, either naturally, or surgically (through removal of your uterus and ovaries), you may decide to go on **Hormone Replacement Therapy (HRT)**.

If you still have your uterus, HRT, like the natural hormones it replaces, can stimulate fibroid growth. More natural herbal supplements, such as RemiFemin (black cohosh), while not as strong, may also have a stimulating effect. If you have fibroids at this stage in your life, and are taking HRT or herbal supplements, it is important to have regular doctors' appointments to monitor your uterus. If you elect to have your reproductive organs removed in a hysterectomy, this will not be an issue. (We'll review hysterectomies in detail in Month 11).

IN A SENTENCE:

> *When you're considering drug treatments, your choice will depend on your age and life goals.*

learning

Drug Therapy

THERE ARE different delivery systems for each drug, meaning some are taken orally, while others are injected or even come in the form of a nasal spray. However you take them, the effects of all these drugs are temporary—which means that the benefits last only as long as you use them. Most of the side effects are temporary too, though there is some debate about whether such treatments as GnRH agonists have long-term side effects on the body after you stop taking them.

Overall, drug therapy seems to be successful in reducing fibroid growth or symptoms for one woman in three (35 percent). Even so, it may be worth exploring prior to trying more invasive solutions, such as surgery. Talk to your doctor about whether any of these drug therapies are right for you, taking into account your symptoms, stage of life, and tolerance for taking medications.

- ○ NSAIDs
- ○ Oral contraceptives (the Pill)
- ○ Levonorgestrel, released from an IUD
- ○ Mifepristone (RU-486)
- ○ GnRH agonists
- ○ Hormone Replacement Therapy (HRT)

NSAIDs

"Non-steroidal anti-inflammatory drugs" is a complicated name for a group of common items: aspirin and over-the-counter drugs known (generically) as ibuprofen and naproxen. As we saw on Day 6, these common remedies can help control cramps and bleeding by either slowing down the production of prostaglandins, which cause pain, or by lowering estrogen levels. If you need to take NSAIDs every day, or if you have very painful cramps or heavy bleeding, talk to your doctor.

The Pill

Nobody really has a definite answer on how—or whether—birth control pills affect fibroids. A 1998 article in *Contraception* magazine said that "Published data on the relationship between fibroids and oral contraceptives appear too scattered to allow a precise quantification of risk"; in August 2000 the American College of Obstetricians and Gynecologists confirmed that "decisions about prescribing oral contraceptives may be complicated" for women with "such underlying conditions . . . as fibroids."

When the Pill was first introduced in 1960, it contained up to 175 micrograms of synthetic estrogen and ten milligrams of synthetic progestin. More recent formulations use as little as twenty micrograms of synthetic estrogen, combined with between 0.15 and 2.5 milligrams of synthetic progestin. This low formulation is still effective at preventing pregnancy, while having fewer long-term side effects.

In the best-case scenario for fibroids, the low estrogen levels in these pills may stop fibroids from growing; this could be because the Pill replaces your normal estrogen and progesterone in smaller amounts than your body would normally produce (see Week 2 for more about estrogen and progesterone). Some doctors believe that women with fibroids are "important candidates" for oral contraceptives. Studies show that the Pill can help reduce heavy bleeding, cramps, and anemia; even the lowest dose pills have been proven to normalize menstrual cycles in 64–82 percent of women who were bleeding between their periods.

On the other hand, the Pill may make fibroids grow more: the National Institutes of Health acknowledge that sometimes the pill can make fibroids worse. If your fibroids have a sudden growth spurt, or if you have pain or tenderness, you should talk to your doctor about going off the Pill.

Some of the different effects of the Pill may be explained by each woman's individual body chemistry and life stage, as we discussed earlier in this chapter as well as in Week 2. If you're in perimenopause, for instance, the amount of estrogen your ovaries produce shifts back and forth, from normal amounts to high amounts to none at all. At this time of life, the Pill can even out your hormones and help prevent the problems caused by fluctuating hormone levels.

One possible idea is to ask your doctor for a blood test which will provide a reading of your estrogen levels. Ideally, you might have this test done several times in the course of one menstrual cycle (such as the beginning, middle, and end) to determine your own levels of natural estrogen. Comparing the amount of your natural estrogen to the amount you would take in the birth control pill might help you and your doctor determine if this is the right solution for you.

Obviously taking the Pill has a number of benefits, not least of which is birth control. If you're on the Pill now, or are considering it, talk to your doctor about the lowest estrogen options, and monitoring your fibroids on a regular basis.

Levonorgestrel-releasing IUDs

Intrauterine devices(IUDs) are another contraception method that may have a side benefit of treating fibroid symptoms, notably, heavy bleeding. In a study of 236 women in Finland, an IUD that released **levonorgestrel** (a synthetic progesterone) effectively reduced heavy bleeding in 80 percent of the women who used it. A very small study, in Poland, looked at the effect of a similar device in women who had fibroids: bleeding was reduced in eleven of the twelve women studied, and their fibroids did not grow in

Danazol (Danocrine) is an androgen, a drug that's chemically similar to the male sex hormone testosterone; it may be prescribed to stop heavy menstrual bleeding caused by a fibroid. The side effects aren't pleasant: they include an increase of male characteristics, such as growing facial hair and making your voice deeper.

the six months after the IUDs were inserted. While IUD therapy seems to be effective in treating heavy bleeding, you should continue to monitor your fibroids for future growth.

Mifepristone (RU-486)

RU-486, the so-called "abortion pill" and "morning-after pill," may also be an effective, if temporary, treatment for fibroids. RU-486, more properly known as **mifepristone**, works by suppressing your natural progesterone, which in turn, as we saw in Week 2, helps suppress fibroid growth.

In 1994, doctors at the University of California, San Diego, found that a twelve-week course of mifepristone reduced fibroids by almost 50 percent—without depriving the women of their natural estrogen. Mifepristone was almost twice as effective as **Lupron** (Lupron Depot®), a GnRH agonist (see the following section), in reducing both uterine artery blood flow and uterine volume.

More recently, a small study at the University of Rochester School of Medicine also showed that mifepristone shrank fibroids up to 50 percent after two months of use; the side effects were limited to mild hot flashes. While this study is far too small to be considered definitive, it helps indicate the potential for this drug to provide temporary—or possibly longer—relief of painful fibroid symptoms. Plans are underway for larger studies, along with an exploration of the longer-term effects of mifepristone, such as whether fibroids grow back, or maintain their reduced size.

Depending on the results of these studies, mifepristone could potentially replace GnRH agonists over time, offering similar benefits with fewer side effects (see below). Ironically, given the controversy over mifepristone's role as an abortion agent, it could even help some women whose fibroids are causing infertility—by shrinking fibroids enough to make pregnancy a possibility after the treatment ends.

GnRH agonists

Short for "gonadotropin releasing hormone," GnRH appears in your body naturally; it's a messenger hormone that tells your body to make estrogen. GnRH agonists are able to block out your natural GnRH and keep

your body from producing estrogen. The technical term for this—truly—
is "chemical castration."

When GnRH agonists shut down your natural production of estrogen,
they create a temporary menopause. The absence of your natural hormones
will usually cause your fibroids to shrink, although the effects only last as
long as you're taking the drug. One large study of women treated with
GnRH agonists for twenty weeks showed that the drug reduced fibroids an
average of 63 percent. One important caveat: the drug was only effective
on sessile fibroids located in the wall of the uterus; pedunculated fibroids
(those hanging on a stalk), and degenerated fibroids did not shrink.

> **THE FDA** has approved Lupron primarily for treating endometriosis and
> prostate cancer; Lupron is also approved for reducing anemia before fibroid sur-
> gery. Using GnRH agonists to shrink fibroids is considered "off label," that is, using
> the drug for conditions other than those officially approved by the FDA. The FDA
> has long allowed doctors a certain amount of discretion in prescribing drugs for
> off-label uses. The Physician's Desk Reference(PDR) even includes an off-label
> guide for treating nearly 1,000 conditions. However, advocacy groups question
> whether we should use drugs as strong as GnRH agonists in ways the FDA hasn't
> adequately tested.

The most common brand name of GnRH agonists is Lupron; other
brand names include Synarel® and Zoladex®. They're not identical—
Lupron is the strongest, with the most extreme side effects—and they are
taken differently, either as a nasal spray, an injection, or monthly implants.
Ask your doctor not just about recommended doses, but about minimum
doses, which can sometimes be equally effective in reducing the size of
fibroids.

There are three primary reasons that your doctor may discuss prescribing GnRH agonists:

If you're perimenopausal, and your fibroids are painful or causing other
symptoms, a course of GnRH agonists may give you relief before the natural effects of menopause take over to reduce the estrogen in your body.

If you're planning to have surgery, your doctor may suggest that you
take GnRH agonists for 1–3 months to shrink the fibroids; the idea is that

your fibroids will be smaller by the time you have the operation, and theoretically, easier to remove. Since GnRH treatment can also cut down bleeding, some doctors prescribe them to make surgery shorter and easier, with less blood loss and less possibility of transfusion. Shrinking your fibroids before surgery may also mean that you can choose a procedure that's easier on your body, with a smaller scar and a shorter stay in the hospital.

However, not every doctor recommends using GnRH agonists before surgery. In some cases, this is because of the number of women who find the side effects extremely difficult to handle; we'll cover those effects shortly. Also, while fibroids are normally firm and well-defined, making them relatively easy to identify and scoop out of your uterus, GnRH agonists make fibroids mushy and harder to remove. Using GnRH agonists can be one of the reasons fibroids "grow back" after myomectomy: they may make some fibroids so small that they're missed during surgery, only to grow again later.

To help treat infertility. Some doctors like to use GnRH agonists instead of surgery if fibroids seem to be preventing pregnancy. The advantage is that even a temporary shrinkage of your fibroids may give you a window to try conceiving without having to recover from surgery and without the potential weakened uterus that surgery can leave behind. If your doctor thinks that fibroids may be causing infertility, three months of taking GnRH agonists may shrink the offending fibroids enough to allow for conception.

For the same reason, GnRH agonists are typically used before **In-Vitro Fertilization (IVF)** to shrink fibroids before implantation. It may make a difference; one study showed that women with untreated intramural and submucosal fibroids (fibroids in the wall or uterine lining) had a much lower rate of success with IVF. Subserosal fibroids—the ones on or near the outer wall of the uterus—are least likely to affect IVF.

While you can't get pregnant while you're in "menopause," the idea is to start trying after you finish the GnRH treatment. If you haven't conceived within 3–6 months or so, your fibroids are likely to come back (though not necessarily in exactly the same position).

There is some evidence that GnRH agonists, either alone or before a surgical treatment such as myomectomy, can restore fertility in some women. In one study of women treated with GnRH agonists and myomectomy, fully 88 percent carried their babies to term. Doctors also perform myomectomies without using GnRH first; you can read more about this topic in Month 10.

It's important to be aware of the potential side effects of GnRH agonists. GnRH agonists deprive your body of estrogen for as long as you take the drug (the typical amount of time that you can expect to be on GnRH agonists, if you choose to take them, is three months, but not more than six to nine months). There are a number of common side effects caused by the low estrogen in your body; your own reaction might be mild or very severe. The most common side effects include:

- hot flashes
- lower sex drive
- vaginal dryness
- bone loss
- weight gain and bloating
- depression
- possible severe pain, resulting from the rapid shrinking of fibroids
- possible increase in cholesterol levels
- possible increased risk of coronary artery disease.

One of the more serious side effects is the loss of bone mineral, which can lead to **osteoporosis**. The decrease might not be reversible; in some studies, bone loss continued for as long as a year after the treatment was finished. (This is why the FDA generally limits any use of GnRH agonists to six months.)

YOU CAN help counter loss of bone density by taking 1500 milligrams of calcium every day and doing weight-bearing exercise. Taking a test called a *Bone Mass Indicator (BMI)* before your treatment will give you a baseline measurement of your bone density; doing it again afterwards will help you see if you actually did suffer any bone loss. Your doctor can refer you to a radiologist for a BMI. The test is quick and simple. The whole procedure takes about five minutes and you don't even have to change out of your street clothes.

As soon as you stop taking GnRH agonists, your fibroids will most likely start growing again. Most studies report that both fibroids and the uterus regain their pre-treatment size within 3–6 months after ending GnRH therapy. One study did show a permanent effect: In the Netherlands, doctors following a group of patients after GnRH treatment found that 40 percent of the women remained symptom free up to five years later.

There is also some controversy about whether the side effects of GnRH agonists are temporary. While many doctors think that side effects vanish when GnRH use stops, women belonging to The National Lupron Victims' Network report that in their own experience the side effects of GnRH can be permanent, and in some cases debilitating. We don't know whether the percentage of women experiencing these problems is large or small; it probably makes sense to consider long-term side effects a possible, if relatively unlikely, outcome of GnRH therapy.

HRT

After we stop ovulating, our ovaries continue to produce a small amount of estrogen, about 10 percent of premenopause levels. Once estrogen levels have dropped this far, the smallest fibroids might disappear, while larger ones don't grow and sometimes even shrink.

At least half of all American women take some form of prescription hormone replacement therapy (HRT) after menopause. If you are considering HRT and still have your uterus—and fibroids—you have to do your homework carefully.

According to *Dr. Susan Love's Hormone Book*, HRT can "reactivate" submucosal fibroids, causing bleeding problems. Dr. Love also points out a study which found that how you take HRT could make a difference; for example, fibroids got bigger "in women using the patch . . . but not in those taking estrogen and a progestin by mouth."

In addition to risks associated with your fibroids, you may have other conditions, such as a family history of breast cancer, that might make you decide not to take HRT.

If you decide to take either a synthetic or natural form of hormone replacement, talk to your doctor about how often you should get a checkup. At a minimum, doctors suggest one exam per year, including a sonogram, to measure your fibroids and check for any precancerous changes.

There are several categories of hormone replacement:

- ○ Natural hormone replacement
- ○ Estrogen replacement therapy
- ○ Hormone replacement therapy
- ○ SERMs

"Natural" hormone replacement. As we reviewed on Day 5 and Week 2, there are a number of herbs and other plants that contain a weak form of estrogen (known as phytoestrogens) that you can eat, take as teas, or use as supplements. The problem with this "natural" hormone replacement is that there's no way to know exactly how much estrogen is getting into your system: the estrogenic effect of foods depends on how much you eat and the quality of the ingredients, and as we saw, the market for teas and supplements is not regulated. Some supplements, such as those containing the herb black cohosh, may replace your estrogen to such a degree that they can also make your fibroids grow. As a result, it's important to work with a qualified practitioner for herbal HRT.

Estrogen Replacement Therapy (ERT). Women who have fibroids are generally warned against taking estrogen alone. For instance, Estrace® (made by Mead Johnson), is a popular drug made from a synthetic form of estradiol, the most potent of our natural estrogens. In laboratory experiments, Estrace® created uterine growth in rats; the instructions for use say that Estrace "should not be administered to patients with leiomyoma of the uterus" (among a number of other conditions) because fibroids "may increase in size during estrogen use." Sudden enlargement, pain, or tenderness of fibroids "requires discontinuation of medication."

Premarin®, made by Wyeth-Ayerst, is another estrogen replacement which, as recently as 1998, was also the most popular form of HRT in the country. There are objections by animal rights groups to how Premarin is made—by repeatedly inducing pregnancies in mares to collect estrogens from their urine—which some women may wish to consider before taking the drug. The "contra-indications" for Premarin include—you guessed it—uterine fibroids.

As you might expect with something as intimate and individual as estrogen, women with fibroids who decide to take it have different experiences:

Some have slow increases in the size of their fibroids, or intermittent bleeding, while others see little or no change at all. Women who take estrogen are three to five times more likely to develop cancer of the uterus than women who do not take estrogen. Of course, if you no longer have your uterus and decide to take ERT, this specific issue won't affect you.

Hormone Replacement Therapy (HRT). This combination of synthetic estrogen and progesterone imitates our natural mix of hormones more than estrogen-only drugs; for that reason, it may be a better bet for women with fibroids. A study reported in *Menopause* notes that a combination of estrogen and progesterone "does not seem to significantly increase uterine or myoma [fibroid] size."

Selective Estrogen Receptor Moderators (SERMs). Also called "designer estrogens," SERMs attempt to send estrogen to the places in your body where it can theoretically do the most good, like your bones, heart, and blood vessels. At the same time, it's supposed to keep estrogen from going to your breasts and uterus, where it can cause problems. As a result of this selectivity, SERMs might seem like a good potential choice for women with fibroids who want to take HRT.

A recent study showed encouraging effects for raloxifene, a SERM marketed as Evista® by Eli Lilly and Co. The drug was tested in Italy on a group of women who still had fibroids after menopause; by the end of raloxifene therapy, fibroids had decreased in size in about 84 percent of the women.

But all the long-term news may not yet be in. SERMs have not been studied extensively enough to know their effects on the various organs of the body. Tamoxifen, for instance, is a SERM used to prevent breast cancer; however, it doubles or triples the risk for uterine cancer. Other SERMs available or in development include droloxifene, idoxifene, and toremifene. If you decide to try a SERM, work closely with your doctor to monitor changes in your body.

Testosterone supplemental therapy for women following hysterectomy can improve sexual libido, sexual pleasure, and sense of well-being. It can also help prevent osteoporosis, and may protect the heart and cardiovascular system.

IN A SENTENCE:

> *Drug therapies temporarily shrink fibroids, or reduce symptoms, but there can be side effects; if you take any form of hormone therapy after menopause, your doctor should continue to monitor you for fibroid growth.*

Fibroids and Pregnancy

FIBROIDS ARE one of the most common conditions among women of childbearing age. This is becoming even more true as women opt to have children after age thirty-five, because while fibroids can affect women of any age, they are most often an issue for women in their thirties and forties.

If you are pregnant, or are planning to conceive, you need not assume that fibroids will automatically cause a problem. Many women who have fibroids have successful pregnancies. However, since fibroids do take up space in your uterus, and may even create a different chemical climate in the uterine cavity, they can have an effect on everything from conception to delivery.

Many women diagnosed with fibroids want to maintain the option of having (more) children, but are just not ready to get pregnant when their fibroids are found. If you have small fibroids, some doctors will suggest that you try to get pregnant as soon as possible, before the fibroids get larger and require treatment or prevent pregnancy.

Only you and your partner can judge your situation and decide if you are ready to start a family, but remember that while fibroids can prevent pregnancy, they don't always. In Month 4 we looked at how drug therapy can shrink fibroids enough to provide a window of opportunity for conception when the therapy ends. In Months 9 and 10, you'll read about medical procedures that can often prolong your fertility by removing or shrinking your fibroids—and let you and your partner prepare to have the family you want, when you are ready.

If you are trying to conceive, and have not been successful so far, it's important to rule out fibroids as a possible cause. In studies of women who have fibroids, there's a high rate of infertility and spontaneous abortion. In particular, fibroids in the uterine cavity (submucous), and in the wall (submural) can have an impact on pregnancy. But there are other conditions that also need to be ruled out, including endometriosis, **salpingitis** (an infection of the Fallopian tubes), and your partner's or donor's fertility.

If you are trying to conceive using In-Vitro Fertilization (IVF), fibroids can lower your chance of successful implantation and pregnancy. In an Australian study, fibroids on the outer wall (subserous) did not affect the success of IVF, but, as in "normal" conception, submucous and submural fibroids presented a problem. In the study, women with these types of fibroids had pregnancy rates of 16 percent and 10 percent after IVF treatment, versus a success rate of over 30 percent for women with either subserous fibroids or no fibroids at all. The authors of this study suggest considering treatment, such as a three to six month course of GnRH agonists (see Month 4), or myomectomy (see Month 10), to shrink or remove fibroids in the uterine wall or cavity before starting IVF. However, another study suggests that if your fibroids are small (under seven centimeters), and don't distort the shape of the uterine cavity, your chances of successful IVF are only slightly less than women with no fibroids.

If you're already pregnant, there's only about a 10 percent chance that your fibroids could cause serious problems: 90 percent of pregnant women with fibroids have either no problems or minor effects. A more frequent side effect of fibroids in pregnancy is psychological distress. While some women are able to stay calm and collected when they hear they've got fibroids, others spend nine months fearing the worst.

Of course, some women do have experiences none of us would wish for, and as with any part of life, there are no guarantees. But as you read about the problems fibroids can create during pregnancy, remember that the most likely outcome is a full-term pregnancy and the birth of a healthy new son or daughter.

Maintain a Pregnancy File

MAINTAINING YOUR own health file during your pregnancy can save time, money, and confusion, especially if you go for second opinions or if for some reason you have to change doctors midway through your pregnancy. Each time you have an appointment, ask your doctor's office to send you copies of every report. If you're keeping a pregnancy log, jot down each appointment, test, and result there. See Week 4 for tips on creating a medical history.

IN A SENTENCE:

Fibroids can complicate pregnancy in several ways, but most women with fibroids have successful pregnancies.

learning

How Can Fibroids Complicate Pregnancy?

MOST FIBROID pregnancies result in happy, healthy babies. But since it is important to be aware of the complications fibroids can cause in pregnancy, this section will outline the possible problems you might face from conception through delivery. Should you feel or notice any unusual symptoms during pregnancy, this information should help you identify any possible problems and know which questions to discuss with your doctor. Be prepared, be aware, but if you can, try not to worry about what "might" happen.

Possible complications fibroids can cause in conception

There are several ways in which fibroids could interfere with your ability to get pregnant:

❍ If you're bleeding continuously, not only is sex less appealing, but the flow of menstrual blood can prevent conception.

❍ If fibroids are blocking one or both Fallopian tubes, they may prevent eggs from entering the uterus. One rare but possible result of this is **ectopic pregnancy**, a dangerous situation in which a fertilized egg begins developing in a Fallopian tube.

○ Fibroids in the uterine wall (submural) may change the uterine lining from a warm, inviting bed to a smooth, hard surface, making it difficult for a fertilized egg to attach to the uterine wall.

○ Fibroids can release chemicals called prostaglandins, a hormone that causes uterine contractions, which can prevent a fertilized egg from landing in the uterine lining.

○ Fibroids can trigger a response from your immune system, sending the body's natural defenses to try to deal with the perceived invader. This reaction is bad news for another "alien" in your body—your fertilized egg.

There are several tests that you can take to rule out—or determine— whether fibroids are the cause of your infertility. These include ultrasound or MRI, **hysterosalpingogram (HSG)** and office **hysteroscopy** (see Month 6 for a full description of these tests).

○ Ultrasound can usually tell you whether your fibroids are inside the cavity or changing the wall of the uterus. MRI can provide a more precise view.

○ A hysterosalpingogram (HSG) can help determine if fibroids are blocking or constricting your Fallopian tubes. Remember, you only need one tube to be open to release an egg, so fibroids would have to be blocking both. HSGs are not always precise: about one in every five tests are wrong, showing a blockage where none exists. This is known as a "false positive." If your HSG shows two blocked tubes, you may want to confirm the diagnosis with a second HSG taken at another time.

○ Hysteroscopy lets your doctor see whether the fibroid is affecting the uterine lining.

If you've been watching your fibroids and trying unsuccessfully to get pregnant for more than twelve months, it may be time to explore stronger options, possibly including drug therapy with GnRH agonists (Month 4) or myomectomy (Month 10).

Possible complications fibroids can cause during pregnancy

- ○ Miscarriage
- ○ Bleeding
- ○ Carneous (Red) Degeneration
- ○ Uterine Crowding
- ○ Placenta Previa
- ○ Placental Abruption
- ○ Premature Rupture of the Membranes (PROM) and Uterine Rupture.

MISCARRIAGE

Having fibroids during a pregnancy does not mean you're automatically at risk for a miscarriage. The fibroids most likely to affect your pregnancy are large, either inside the uterine cavity or wall. Multiple fibroids that are big enough to enlarge your uterus can also put you more at risk. (Fibroids are not the only reason women miscarry, of course: 15–30 percent of U.S. women have miscarriages every year.)

Fibroids can cause miscarriage in four primary ways, by:

- ○ distorting the uterine cavity;
- ○ competing with the growing fetus for the same blood supply—and winning;
- ○ causing the uterus to contract and expel the embryo, through the release of prostaglandins;
- ○ triggering a response from your immune system, creating an inhospitable climate in the uterus for the growing embryo.

If a fibroid causes a miscarriage, it's more likely to happen in the first or second trimester. Later in pregnancy, fibroids are more likely to cause pain or preterm contractions than miscarriage.

BLEEDING

This is one of the more common effects fibroids can cause during pregnancy. Depending on how far along your pregnancy is, bleeding can signal different problems; The American Nurses Association (ANA) recommends that you call your doctor for any vaginal bleeding during pregnancy. Slight bleeding or spotting can be normal, especially in the first trimester.

Carneous (red) degeneration

This is the term used for fibroids that degenerate during pregnancy. If you remember from Day 1, "degeneration" describes what happens when fibroids outgrow their blood supply and begin to die. **Carneous (red) degeneration** during pregnancy affects about 10 percent of women.

The most common sign of red degeneration is pain, most often centered over the fibroid, and usually beginning around twenty weeks. Other symptoms include pain radiating into your lower back, light bleeding (always a sign to talk to your doctor during pregnancy), nausea, vomiting, or low-grade fever.

The pain of red degeneration might be very severe. While you should absolutely call your doctor, keep in mind that degeneration doesn't hurt your baby. The pain may last from a few days to over a week, and many doctors simply suggest bed rest and acetaminophen (such as Tylenol®) or ibuprofen (such as Advil®), though these aren't always strong enough to conquer the pain. If necessary, your doctor can give you a prescription pain reliever; she may also suggest hospitalization, so you can get pain medications and fluids through an IV line. You may need antibiotics if you have a fever or other signs of infection.

A word of caution: please don't self-medicate, even with common pain relievers such as aspirin, acetaminophen, naproxen, or ibuprofen, without speaking to your doctor. For any drugs you take during pregnancy, make sure you ask your doctor about possible side effects, especially any risk of miscarriage.

Uterine crowding

If you already had fibroids before your pregnancy, these can increase three to five times in size; this is a result of the extra hormones your body produces when you're pregnant. Fibroids that take up space inside your uterus can cause uterine crowding: in some women, the effect is almost like carrying twins.

Having a large fibroid pregnancy often means that you'll get bigger sooner, and will often get bigger than you would normally. As a result, symptoms more common in late pregnancy can occur earlier, like back pain, hemorrhoids, varicose veins, difficulty breathing, and heartburn.

The effects on the baby are usually mild. The baby's head and other body parts may look distorted at birth, but in most cases, the passage of time reshapes the body naturally. The most severe—and unusual—possibilities include underdeveloped lungs, a misshapen skull or face, a dislocated hip, bowed legs, or clubfoot.

PLACENTA PREVIA

Normally, the placenta forms at the top of the uterus, the part farthest from the cervix. But if you have fibroids at the top of the uterus, the placenta may form near the cervix. In the third trimester, your cervix begins to expand. If the placenta is near the cervix, it can tear loose, creating a raw spot that bleeds. This is called **placenta previa**; it happens to about one in every 200 pregnant women.

Your doctor can tell where your placenta is using an ultrasound. If your doctor thinks you have placenta previa, you might need to avoid having any more pelvic exams before delivery, as this can make any bleeding worse. You may also need to avoid intercourse for the rest of your pregnancy.

One warning sign for placenta previa is bright red bleeding, starting around the sixth month. Other things to watch out for are pain that comes on suddenly and doesn't go away in the area of your uterus and lower back; a feeling of tenderness in your uterus; or early contractions.

You may have to be confined to bed for the rest of your pregnancy, possibly even in a hospital, and you might need drugs to prevent premature labor. The worst case scenario includes severe bleeding: while painless, it can put you at a greater risk for infection and deprive your baby of adequate oxygen, affecting his growth and development. If your blood loss is severe, you might need a transfusion.

Sometimes the placenta can move again, basically solving the problem on its own. Even so, the majority of women—up to 75 percent—whose placenta shifts in this way will have to have early delivery, generally via C-section. If placenta previa occurs after the thirty-seventh week, and the placenta is not blocking the cervix, you may be able to deliver vaginally.

PLACENTAL ABRUPTION

Normally, the placenta stays attached to the wall of your uterus until your baby is born. Placental abruption is when your placenta separates from the wall of the uterus sometime between the twentieth and thirty-seventh week of your pregnancy. While no one knows the exact cause, fibroids can be one of the suspects.

It's hard to tell whether you have placental abruption, since many of the symptoms are similar to other conditions, including heavy bleeding, contractions, lower back pain, and tenderness in the area of your uterus. Even ultrasound can't always tell exactly what's going on. If your pregnancy is far enough along, your doctor may opt for early delivery, possibly by C-section. At any point in your pregnancy, you should contact your doctor immediately about any unusual symptoms.

It's possible that extra folic acid may help prevent placental abruption; this is a B vitamin that can be found in many B-complex or multivitamin tablets. Talk to your doctor about whether extra folic acid is something that could work for you.

PREMATURE RUPTURE OF THE MEMBRANES (PROM)
AND UTERINE RUPTURE

The extra size of fibroids can put pressure on the flexible but delicate membrane surrounding your unborn baby. In extreme cases, fibroids can cause this membrane to break open, or rupture.

If this happens, some of the **amniotic fluid** will begin to leak. Your first sensation could be a gush of fluid, followed by continuous dripping, like a leaky faucet. This can cause premature delivery and infection, so a prompt call to your doctor or visit to an emergency room is critical. Other warning signs of uterine rupture can include severe pain in your abdomen; you may even feel a sensation of something tearing inside you. You may faint; your heartbeat and breathing may become rapid. Once again, call your doctor or seek emergency care immediately.

If your doctor is concerned about the possibility of rupture, you may find yourself on bed-rest to avoid putting the extra pressure of gravity on your uterus. This, plus close observation by your doctor, will normally protect both you and your baby.

More uncommon is the risk of uterine rupture during labor or early contractions. You're generally only at risk if you've had surgery on your uterus; the scars from a Caesarean, myomectomy, myolysis, or cryomyolysis can weaken your uterus so that it can't withstand the pressure of labor.

Possible complications fibroids can cause during and after delivery

- O Preterm labor
- O C-sections
- O Postpartum hemorrhage

If your fibroids haven't caused a problem so far, you may be able to deliver normally, though this is a subject you'll discuss with your doctor. There's also a possibility that your delivery will be a little different than you'd planned, either because of premature labor, the possibility of needing a C-section, or the danger of bleeding after delivery.

PRETERM LABOR

Preterm deliveries are those that begin anytime between 20–36 weeks, as opposed to the "normal" full-term pregnancy, which occurs at 37–40 weeks. Women with fibroids have a higher risk of preterm labor; your risk is also higher if you're over thirty-five, or have had abdominal surgery.

How will you know if you're going into preterm labor? It may be difficult to tell, but here are some of the warning signs:

- O uterine contractions every fifteen minutes or faster
- O menstrual-like cramps
- O a dull ache in the lower back
- O pressure or a feeling of fullness in your lower abdomen
- O increase or change in vaginal discharge. The fluid may turn pink or brown, and may be either watery or contain more mucus than usual.

If you do go into labor early, bed rest and extra liquids may help stop the contractions. If not, your doctor may suggest a drug called a **tocolytic**. While this is often helpful, the side effects can be unnerving, including headaches, rapid pulse rate, nervousness, dizziness, and shortness of breath.

As for any preemie, the earlier the birth, the more the potential complications, and the more care your child will need. There are no guarantees, but with proper medical attention and care from you, most children born early have a good chance of developing normally.

C-SECTIONS

Not all women with fibroids will need a C-section, but fibroids do increase your likelihood for several reasons:

○ Fibroids in the lower part of your uterus can block the baby's descent.

○ Many fibroids can keep your uterus from contracting properly, preventing progress in labor.

○ If fibroids change the shape of your uterus, they can influence the position of your baby, so that instead of being positioned normally (head down), she could be positioned feet first, in the breech position, or sideways, in the transverse position.

○ If you've already had a Caesarean delivery or myomectomy, the scars might make your body too weak for a normal delivery, but the chances are 50:50 that you can still deliver normally after a previous surgery.

Complications of C-sections for mothers can include infection, excessive bleeding, reaction to a possible transfusion, or reaction to anesthesia. There are fewer dangers to the baby. There is a possibility that general anesthesia given to the mother may affect the baby by reducing its oxygen supply or by depressing the baby's breathing; fortunately, this is rare and can generally be managed successfully.

Fibroids can also be removed during a C-section, in a technique called **Caesarean myomectomy**. One study showed no greater risk of complications from Caesarean myomectomy than a C-section alone.

Interestingly, women often seem to recover much faster from C-sections than from other types of abdominal surgery, possibly because they know their new baby is depending on them, or even because the surgery was for a happy reason rather than to fix a problem. In any case, you will need at least a week of complete recovery time, and experts suggest that you'll recover faster if you don't rush it.

POSTPARTUM HEMORRHAGE

Bleeding is common after delivery, but if you have fibroids, you might have a greater risk. Why? When the placenta separates from the wall of the uterus, the exposed blood vessels bleed freely. Normally, your uterus should contract and shut the vessels off; fibroids can keep that from happening. If you've suffered from placental abruption, premature labor, or uterine rupture as a result of your fibroids, you may also be at risk for postpartum hemorrhage.

If you're bleeding too much after delivery, the first thing your doctor may do is massage your uterus; this can help your uterus contract, shutting off open blood vessels. Your doctor may also inject a drug to slow down the bleeding, pack your uterus with gauze, or tie off the uterine arteries. In extreme cases, your doctor may have to perform a hysterectomy.

If your doctor thinks you may be at risk for excessive bleeding when you deliver, discuss the pros and cons of donating your own blood in advance for a possible transfusion.

IN A SENTENCE:

> *Most of the problems fibroids can cause in pregnancy do not affect the health of the baby.*

MONTH 6

Get a Check-Up

IT'S BEEN six months since you found out you have fibroids. It's time to take inventory, check in with yourself, review your Lifestyle and Symptoms Indicator (Day 3), and see your doctor for a checkup.

To start off, ask yourself these questions:

○ How are your symptoms? Are they better, worse, or the same as they were six months ago? Have you noticed any new symptoms?

○ Have you made any lifestyle changes that might make your fibroid symptoms better? Worse?

○ Have you tried any alternative treatments? What were the results?

○ Have you been using any drug therapies, including aspirin or ibuprofen? Have they helped?

○ Have your periods changed at all, either in how many days they last, or how many days/weeks between periods? Has your bleeding become heavier or lighter?

Answer these questions as honestly as you can, referring to your Lifestyle and Symptoms Indicator, as well as your Menstrual Diary (Week 2) to help refresh your memory of life over the past six months.

You can jot down a few notes to take with you to your next doctor's appointment. If you wish, add them to the top of your medical history (Week 4). Here's a suggested outline for your notes, but they can be in whatever form suits you best.

My fibroids were diagnosed on (*date*)
My symptoms then were (*note heavy, medium, or light for each*):
- ◯ Bleeding
- ◯ Cramps
- ◯ Pain/Pressure
- ◯ Urinary/Bowel problems
- ◯ Fatigue
- ◯ Other: _____

My symptoms as of (*today's date*) are (*note heavy, medium, or light for each*):
- ◯ Bleeding
- ◯ Cramps
- ◯ Pain/Pressure
- ◯ Urinary/Bowel problems
- ◯ Fatigue
- ◯ Other: _____

My symptoms as of (*today's date*) are:
- ◯ Better
- ◯ Worse
- ◯ The same

I've changed my diet by (*note increasing or decreasing for each*):
- ◯ Sugar
- ◯ Fat
- ◯ Full-fat dairy products
- ◯ Low-fat or fat-free dairy products
- ◯ Meat
- ◯ Chicken
- ◯ Fish

O Soy
O Vegetables
O Fruit
O Whole grains

I've changed my lifestyle habits by (*note increasing or decreasing for each*):
O Exercise
O Sleep
O Stress reduction

I've tried alternative therapies (*note with or without symptom reduction*)
O Western herbalism (*note specific herbs or preparations*)
O Chinese herbalism (*note specific herbs or preparations*)
O Acupuncture
O Ayur-Veda
O Naturopathy
O Homeopathy
O Other: _____

I am trying to get pregnant (*yes/no*)
O If yes, I have been trying for _____ (*number of weeks/months/ years*)

Reviewing your answers to this checklist should help you summarize all of the efforts you've made to improve your health and well-being since you were first diagnosed, and help remind you what lifestyle changes and alternative treatments seem to help improve your fibroid symptoms.

When you go to the ob-gyn for your six-month check-up, take this summary with you to discuss with her. This information, plus an examination and a sonogram, will give both you and your doctor the information you need to move forward.

O The best possibility is that your fibroid symptoms are controlled and the methods you've tried so far are working to keep your fibroids manageable. If your doctor agrees this is the case, then you can continue on this course indefinitely, checking in with your doctor every six months to get a thorough physical.

○ If your symptoms seem worse and you have not tried changing your diet, exercise, or other habits, and if you have not tried alternative therapies, you still can, assuming your symptoms haven't become too serious or your fibroids very large.

○ If, however, your symptoms seem worse and you have tried making changes, you may need to consider conventional medical treatments. As you'll see in the following chapters, there are many options available to treat fibroids. After you've read about them, and done your homework, one of them will feel right to you. Remember, choosing medical treatment, if you need it, is also part of taking care of yourself.

IN A SENTENCE:

> *No matter what your fibroid symptoms are, scheduling a check-up with your doctor every six months is an important way of taking care of yourself.*

Other Tests
You May Need

YOUR CHECK-UP will most likely include a thorough physical exam in your doctor's office, including a **Pap smear**. Your doctor should also send you for a sonogram to determine if your fibroids have grown since your first diagnosis (see Day 2 if you'd like a refresher on sonograms).

If your fibroids seem to have grown, if your symptoms have gotten noticeably worse, or if you are having problems trying to conceive, your doctor may recommend one or more of the following tests.

- Complete Blood Count (CBC)
- Magnetic Resonance Imaging (MRI)
- Hysterosalpingogram (HSG)
- Hysteroscopy
- Laparoscopy

Complete Blood Count (CBC)

One short stab in the arm with a hypodermic needle can usually draw enough blood to perform a CBC, or Complete

Blood Count, also known as "taking bloods." If you're having heavy bleeding, or are scheduled for any kind of surgery, a CBC can show if you have anemia. In addition, a test called a **Coagulation Profile** can rule out von Willebrand's disease. Both anemia and von Willebrand's are discussed on Day 3.

Since about 5 percent of healthy people get abnormal or borderline values on lab tests, it's important to get an experienced second opinion before proceeding with any radical treatment based on one blood test.

Magnetic Resonance Imaging (MRI)

Magnetic Resonance Imaging (MRI) goes a step beyond sonograms in picturing your uterus and ovaries (see Day 2 for a complete description of sonograms). Sonograms tend to be fairly accurate, but if you're contemplating invasive therapy for your fibroids, such as surgery, an MRI can provide a more precise picture due to its ability to provide greater details of soft tissue and fluids.

MRIs can supplement the information gained from sonograms by:

○ providing a better image of the ovaries when fibroids are present.
○ detecting masses in the uterus that might be missed by a sonogram.
○ showing the position of the dominant fibroid within the uterus, which can help to determine which type of treatment is most appropriate.
○ distinguishing adenomyosis (see Day 3) from fibroids more accurately.

MRI uses large, powerful magnets to energize subatomic particles in your body. The bigger the machine, the more expensive the magnets are, so if you think the opening will be as small and narrow as possible, you're right. For some women, MRIs are no big deal, but others find it can be unpleasant.

You will have to change into a hospital gown and slippers before this procedure. (If your feet tend to get cold, bring socks or slippers from home, just in case they are not provided.) You'll be led into a room with a large machine; you'll see a technician behind a glass wall who will be in voice contact with you during the procedure.

You'll be helped onto a sort of tray, which is then slid—with you on it—into a large tube. If you're concerned about your reaction to being in an enclosed space, talk to your doctor about the possibility of having conscious sedation or even anesthesia. Both of these are used to help patients get through the test with as little discomfort as possible. Some newer MRIs are open, meaning that you don't have to go through the darkness of lying in the tube; however, since these open machines are less powerful, the scans can take twice as long to complete.

An MRI is painless. But during the test, you'll hear bursts of horrific noise, like a jackhammer: this is the action of the magnets at work. A relaxed attitude will be your best protection against the difficulties of this test. The worst hardship—assuming your insurance is covering the extremely high cost—is the fear that the strange MRI environment can create.

Hysterosalpingogram (HSG)

This is yet another way to take a picture of your uterus, this time using X-rays. If you're trying to get pregnant, hysterosalpingograms (HSG) offer one important advantage over sonograms: they can help tell you if your Fallopian tubes are open or blocked by fibroids.

You should not have an HSG if there's any chance that you're already pregnant, since it can harm an embryo or fetus. You should also avoid the test if you've got undiagnosed vaginal bleeding, pelvic inflammatory disease (PID), or if you're menstruating. Tell your doctor if you're allergic to any medications or to the dyes used for the X-ray.

The test will most likely take place at a radiologist's office, generally someone recommended by your gynecologist. You'll undress either all the way or from the waist down, just as you do for a pelvic exam.

Since this procedure can hurt, some doctors will give you a non-steroidal anti-inflammatory drug such as Aleve® or Motrin® before the procedure; some may give you a local anesthetic, although in fairness, the shot that delivers the anesthetic can hurt almost as much as the procedure itself. If you're concerned about the possibility of pain, call the radiologist's office and talk with him or her in advance.

While you're lying on a table with your feet in stirrups, the doctor will clamp your cervix open with a special forceps called a **tenaculum**. Using a syringe, the doctor will slowly pour an opaque dye into your uterus. The dye creates a picture on the developed X-ray film, showing your uterus, Fallopian tubes, and ovaries, as well as any abnormalities in the shape or lining of the uterus and any obstructions blocking your Fallopian tubes. An HSG does not necessarily show fibroids deep in the uterine wall (intramural) or fibroids on the outside of the uterus (subserosal).

Cramps after the test are considered normal; if they continue for more than a day or so, call your doctor. Other complications can include bleeding, infection, or allergic reaction to the dye, which can show up as hives, itching, or low blood pressure.

> **BEFORE YOU** take any test more invasive than a sonogram or CBC, you'll need to sign a consent form. Amber Wood, R.N., says "a consent form is necessary before any operation, or even any test procedure. This is how you give your permission to perform the work you and your doctor have agreed to."

Hysteroscopy

This procedure gives your doctor direct visual access to the inside of your uterus without surgery. **Hysteroscopy** is used both to get a diagnosis as well as to perform surgery on the uterine lining.

A diagnostic hysteroscopy can be done in your doctor's office; your doctor can even take a small tissue sample (a **biopsy**) at the same time. For a diagnostic hysteroscopy, a tiny, thin, lighted telescope is inserted into your vagina, allowing your doctor to get an insider's view of your uterus, including the entrance to your Fallopian tubes—a crucial area to check if you're trying to get pregnant.

Hysteroscopy can also be used to remove fibroids inside the uterine cavity (submucosal); this is known as surgical hysteroscopy, or hysteroscopy and resection. Because of the greater risks involved in a surgical procedure, this operation is best done in a hospital setting. A hysteroscopy cannot remove fibroids in the wall or on the outer wall of the uterus. We'll discuss surgical hysteroscopy in more detail in Month 10.

Hysteroscopy is generally done with local anesthesia, but as we said in the discussion on HSG, an injection of a local anesthesia in the cervix can be more painful than the procedure itself. In response to what some

women call "intolerable pain," doctors have developed a two-step procedure, using a lidocaine spray to numb the cervix before the injection. In a
study of 300 women, this two-step method made a significant difference,
allowing many of the women having the test to have a more comfortable
experience.

There are three potential complications you should know about:

○ Perforation of the uterus. While the uterus usually heals quickly,
  scarring could be a potential problem if you're considering pregnancy.
○ Fluid leaking into your bloodstream. Your doctor may use a saline
  solution or other fluid to enlarge your uterus to get a more precise
  view. Sometimes, some of this fluid can leak into the blood vessels
  of the uterus: too much fluid in your blood vessels can cause fluid
  on the lungs (pulmonary edema) or even seizures. As a rule, this is
  prevented by keeping track of the amount of fluid used during the
  procedure. For more about avoiding this particular complication, see
  the section on surgical hysteroscopy in Month 10.
○ Bleeding. A little spotting afterwards is normal, but if you're bleeding heavily, call your doctor immediately.

Laparoscopy

This is a somewhat more invasive way for your doctor to get a firsthand
look at you. By putting a tiny camera directly into your abdomen, your doctor can see the outside of your uterus as well as the surrounding pelvic
structure. **Laparoscopy** can be combined with a hysteroscopy to see what's
happening inside your uterus, or with a **D&C** to take a sample of the tissue inside your uterus (see Month 7 for more about D&C).

Laparoscopies are almost always done in a hospital, though on an outpatient basis, meaning you won't have to stay overnight. You may be surprised to learn that the first laparoscopy on a human being was done as
recently as 1987. As a result, not every doctor is an expert in the technique.
Before you commit to surgery, ask your doctor about his experience doing
laparoscopy and make sure he is Board-certified. If you have any doubts,
or just want reassurance, ask to talk to some other patients who've had a
laparoscopy with him.

If your doctor detects any problems during the laparoscopy, she may want to perform surgery right then and there. Depending on your condition, this may be a good, efficient option, but only you can decide if you are comfortable trusting your doctor's judgment during surgery or if you want to have a further conversation before she does anything more than take a look inside. Have a conversation with your doctor before you have the procedure about the possibility of surgery during this test, and come to an agreement about what you will and will not permit.

The day before your laparoscopy, you won't be able to eat or drink anything for twelve hours; if you can schedule the test for the morning, you can minimize your fasting time. When you arrive at the hospital, you'll be given a locker for your clothing and handbag or other personal items. It's wise not to bring any valuables or jewelry to the hospital. You'll change into a hospital gown, robe, and slippers, and you'll be issued a little plastic shower cap for the operating room. A nurse or physician's assistant will take your medical history and blood pressure.

Laparoscopies can be performed with either local or general anesthesia; some doctors will start with a local and only move on to general anesthesia if they find a potential problem they need to explore more thoroughly. Of course, if you know of any allergies you have to anesthesia, be sure you tell your doctor, the hospital staff, and the anesthesiologist. If you're getting a local anesthetic, you'll be awake during the surgery, but you shouldn't feel anything after the injection of the anesthetic. The injection can hurt—ask if the doctor will numb the area first. If you're having general anesthesia, you'll fall asleep almost instantly and not feel a thing until you wake up in the recovery room.

Once you're prepped for surgery, your doctor will make two small cuts inside your belly button, about 1–2 cm long. Using a needle, the doctor will fill your uterus with gas—carbon dioxide, or CO_2—which distends your uterus and makes it taut. Carbon dioxide is easily absorbed by the blood. For younger, otherwise healthy women, the most common effect of CO_2 is nausea. You may also experience an odd pain in your shoulder, or some lingering abdominal pain. In some cases, mostly involving older women, carbon dioxide puts pressure on the blood vessels and heart, creating a slight danger of having a stroke.

The more severe, but unusual, surgical risks of laparoscopy include perforating a blood vessel, the bowel, or liver. Your risk of complications will be higher than normal if you suffer from obesity, heart, or lung disease, if you smoke, are in the late stages of pregnancy, or if you take certain medications, including antihypertensives, antiarrhythmics, diuretics, or beta-adrenagic blockers.

When the surgery is over, your doctor will close the incision with small sutures or staples, and put a small bandage over the wound. You'll rest in the hospital for a few hours to make sure your vital signs are all in order. Someone will need to accompany you home even if you live in a big city and can take a cab or mass transit; you will not usually be allowed to drive home yourself.

Most women recover from a laparoscopic test within a day or two. Don't drink anything carbonated—soda, seltzer, beer, champagne—for two days after surgery. The carbon dioxide still in your system can interact with these drinks, causing vomiting. Call your doctor immediately if you start showing signs of infection: headache, muscle pain, dizziness, or fever, if you start bleeding a lot from either the incision or your vagina, or if you have abdominal swelling or pain.

IN A SENTENCE:

> *There is a wide range of tests available to picture your uterus and fibroids, which can help determine what kind of treatment, if any, is appropriate for you.*

HALF-YEAR MILESTONE

Now that you're halfway through your first year with fibroids, you've explored all the ways you can live with fibroids without having surgery, by:

- ○ **LEARNING HOW TO HANDLE FIBROID-RELATED "BLUES."**

- ○ **UNDERSTANDING HOW FIBROIDS CAN AFFECT BOTH SEX AND PREGNANCY.**

- ○ **EXPLORING ALTERNATIVE TREATMENTS FOR FIBROIDS AND SYMPTOMS, SUCH AS ACUPUNCTURE AND HERBALISM.**

- ○ **LEARNING HOW CERTAIN DRUGS CAN HELP YOU MANAGE YOUR FIBROIDS.**

As you now enter the last half of the year, you can learn more about the variety of medical techniques that you can explore, if you choose to, including:

- ○ **UTERINE ARTERY EMBOLIZATION (UAE).**

- ○ **MYOMECTOMY.**

- ○ **HYSTERECTOMY.**

You'll also read about how to find a specialist, preparing for surgery, and recovering and staying healthy.

Choosing a Doctor for Special Treatments

IF YOU'VE decided that you need or want invasive medical treatment for your fibroids, you need to think carefully about your choice of doctors. Your current ob-gyn may be the right person for you, but in some cases, you may decide that you want to find a doctor with different skills for surgery.

Not every doctor does every procedure, or is equally skilled in every procedure. For instance, if you opt to have Uterine Artery Embolization (Month 9), that procedure is not done by an ob/gyn at all, but by a specialist called an interventional radiologist. Similarly, only about 10 percent of ob-gyns perform the surgery called hysteroscopic resections. Whether you decide to stick with your current physician or look for someone new, there are several issues that you should consider.

Experience. For any procedure, be sure to ask your doctor about his or her experience. Find out how long your doctor has been performing the kind of treatment he or she is recommending, and how many procedures he or she has actually done.

Your doctor should be Board-certified as well as have advanced training in specialties such as laparoscopy, hysteroscopy, or interventional radiology, depending on the procedure they are offering you.

If you decide to seek out a specialist—whether in UAE, myomectomy, or any other procedure—bear in mind that these doctors have made a huge professional commitment to the type of surgery they practice. Don't necessarily expect them to give you a rundown of your other options; use the time in your appointment to learn as much as possible about the doctor you're meeting, and the treatment you're discussing.

Listening skills. A 1984 study found that most doctors interrupted patients eighteen seconds into an interview. Doctors come into your appointment with their own beliefs and experiences: these may or may not be in sync with your own. Some doctors may not understand why you would want to preserve your uterus—others may resist your interest in having your uterus removed. It's very important to feel that your doctor is listening to what you want, and why. In turn, you can learn a lot from listening objectively to your doctor's recommendations and evaluation of all the available options. Remember, you and your doctor will be a team: you must feel that you can work together.

Comfort level. In addition to the intellectual comfort level that comes from knowing your doctor is a skilled, accredited, experienced physician, your comfort can be affected by a variety of factors. Most of us want our doctors to have a caring attitude in addition to a high level of expertise: someone who will reassure us about our fears, answer our questions, and accept our less-than-perfect health care routines. The courtesy and professionalism of the office staff can enhance—or detract from—your confidence and feelings of being cared for. Even the decor and location of the office can affect your feeling of well-being. While I wouldn't suggest choosing a doctor based on office decor, this type of observation can give you a clue about a new doctor's personality and work style.

And then there's the delicate question of gender. Can a male doctor understand a woman's body and emotional concerns? While statistics show that male gynecologists are more likely to recommend hysterectomies, younger doctors of both genders are more likely to talk to you about a range of treatment options. A recent survey by the American College of Obstetricians and Gynecologists (ACOG) found that women overall are evenly split in their preferences for male and female physicians, although women under thirty were more likely to prefer talking to a woman gynecologist.

What's most important is to know what your own preference is, if any, for the doctor who will make you feel most comfortable.

Other patients' experiences. One important resource for assessing your potential doctor is his or her other patients. Feel free to ask for a list of women you can talk to—and then call a few of them for a heart-to-heart. While the women on a list like this have most likely had positive experiences, you'll still be able to pick up a lot of clues about the procedure, any side effects, the doctor's bedside manner, and your expected recovery time.

Investigating Malpractice

THE THREAT of malpractice looms for virtually all doctors; the complaints are not always justified, or even true. However, to the extent possible, you should investigate your doctor's record of complaints. A call to your state's Department of Health, or a visit to their website, can help you determine if your doctor has been involved in legal action, and what the outcome was. If you do find evidence of legal action, you should take into account both the type of complaint (i.e., how serious was the act in question), as well as the number of complaints a doctor has received over the course of his or her career.

Be aware that even if a doctor has a history of incompetence or malpractice, he or she may be reprimanded, dismissed, or relieved of hospital privileges—without actually getting sued. These actions don't appear in public records and are notoriously difficult to find out about. Your best bet here is to ask other previous patients whether the doctor has any known history of problems or malpractice suits, especially if your doctor has recently changed hospital affiliations, or has started a new practice.

If your doctor works in a managed care organization, he or she may need a lot of pressure from you to manage your case as thoroughly as necessary. According to a study in the *New England Journal of Medicine*, doctors working for managed care organizations feel they aren't supposed to tell patients about expensive treatments; more than half of the doctors said they were discouraged from referring patients to specialists, which in some cases led to reduced quality of care.

Once you've determined that a doctor is right for you, whether you're seeing a new physician or sticking with your current practitioner, there are specific steps you can take to get the most out of your appointments. Some of these suggestions can also help you have conversations with your current doctor about the procedures you're considering.

○ Make a list of questions and topics you want to discuss and bring it with you to your appointment. It's all right to read your questions to the doctor. And remember, every question you have is valid; there is no such thing as a "stupid" question.

○ Bring two copies of your medical history (Week 4), one for you and one for your doctor, to review together.

○ Bring two copies of your Lifestyle and Symptoms Indicator (Day 3) and your Menstrual Diary (Week 2). This will help keep your conversation focused and factual.

○ Bring along this book, or other books and articles that help you describe your symptoms, the treatment(s) you're considering, or other questions.

○ After the doctor examines you, don't hesitate to ask specific questions about the diagnosis and treatment plan. If something isn't clear, ask your doctor to explain it in less technical language. Keep asking questions until you are comfortable that you understand what has been discussed. (One helpful technique you can use is called "Playback." When the doctor says something that you find unclear or confusing, repeat it back by saying, "I understand you're saying that _____," or "What I hear you saying is _____." The doctor will respond. Continue going back and forth in this way until you're satisfied that you have a complete understanding of what the doctor is recommending.)

○ Wait for test results on any preliminary diagnosis—for anemia, infertility, even bleeding—before making any treatment decisions.

○ Ask your doctor why he or she has recommended the course of action that seems to be his or her preference.

○ Ask your doctor if there are any alternative recommendations he or she would make; this can be useful in seeing how up-to-date or open-minded the doctor is about new or different treatments.
○ If at all possible, bring a friend or relative with you to take notes and remind you to ask the questions on your "cheat sheet."

Of course, be straightforward and polite, and remember, you're there to learn. But don't worry about what your doctor thinks of you. It's much more important to figure out what you think of him or her.

IN A SENTENCE:

> *Your doctor is your healthcare partner; finding someone you trust and respect is an important part of your overall health care.*

learning

Fibroids and Cancer

A NATURAL question you may have is whether fibroids increase your risk of uterine cancer. The prevailing wisdom is that they do not; the National Institutes of Health state firmly that fibroids "are not associated with cancer, they virtually never develop into cancer, and they do not increase a woman's risk for uterine cancer."

However, studies estimate that between 0.1 percent and 1 percent of women with fibroids may get uterine cancer at some point in their lives. That equals 10 to 100 women out of every 10,000, with women over fifty having a statistically greater risk than younger women. These numbers are definitely higher than the statistic offered by the American Cancer Society for uterine cancer among women in general, which is about 0.02 percent, or 2 in every 10,000 women. (Remember, that even using the highest probabilities, of 10,000 women with fibroids, at least 9,900 will not get cancer.)

In cases where women with fibroids do get cancer, doctors don't know if the fibroids themselves become cancerous—especially when they begin to degenerate—or if there's an underlying problem related to both fibroids and cancer. There's no reason to panic or assume the worst, and the odds are very much in your favor. But to play it safe, especially if you've been experiencing rapid growth or abnormal bleeding, your doctor should test you for cancer.

ACCORDING TO the National Cancer Institute, there are three types of cancer that affect the uterus:

○ The most common is endometrial or uterine cancer, which begins in the lining of the uterus, or endometrium.

○ The second type, called uterine sarcoma, starts in the muscles of the uterus. Uterine cancer and uterine sarcoma occur most often during or after menopause—the first sign is unusual bleeding, which may start as a watery flow that gradually contains more blood.

○ The third type of cancer affecting the uterus is cervical cancer: This can be most commonly detected with an annual Pap smear.

Having a test for cancer, based on your symptoms and perhaps family history, does not mean that you have cancer. Before anybody gives you a diagnosis of cancer, they must be able to rule out the benign possibilities. If you are found to have cancer, hysterectomy is considered absolutely necessary, most likely followed by radiation and chemotherapy.

Unfortunately, some doctors recommend hysterectomy to prevent future cancers . . . even when a woman has no current trace of the disease. There's no question that a woman without a uterus can't get uterine cancer, but as you've seen, your statistical risk is low. There are no data supporting the use of "preventive" or **prophylactic surgeries** of any kind in women whose fibroids are not presenting problems . . . while studies are clear that these procedures do have a risk of complications. Unless your family history or other factors suggest you're at risk, you should think long and hard about this type of prophylactic surgery. For most women, the risks involved in surgery are greater than the risk of getting cancer.

On the other hand, some women with both cancer and fibroids report that their original doctors never tested for cancer, assuming instead that their unusual bleeding was due to their fibroids. For this reason, women who have had gynecological cancers strongly recommend seeing a **gynecological oncologist** (a doctor who specializes in women's cancers), to rule out any malignant growths. If you're bleeding in any unusual way and your fibroids are in the uterine wall (intramural) or on the outer wall (subserous), or if you're past menopause, insist on a biopsy: if you have cancer, with luck, a biopsy will catch it early.

If your doctor suspects that there is a problem, there are a range of methods that can be used to test for cancer, from the relatively simple blood test called a CA-125 to an outpatient visit to the hospital for a D&C.

CA-125

This simple blood test is used to help diagnose ovarian cancer. (It is not a "screener" for cancer; as we'll see, having high test results can be caused by a number of benign conditions.) Although fibroids are not related to ovarian cancer, doctors have traditionally expressed concern that large fibroids prevent them from feeling enlarged ovaries in a pelvic exam or seeing them in a sonogram. While newer, high-resolution ultrasound, MRI, or CT scans are helping to resolve part of this problem, a CA-125, in combination with these tests, can help tell you and your doctor if you have a potential problem.

The entire test consists of your doctor drawing blood from your arm, just as she would in any normal blood test. The procedure will be over in seconds. The blood is then sent to a lab for analysis.

The lab will look for something in your blood called a **biochemical tumor marker**. Higher levels of this marker in your blood may indicate the presence of cancer cells. Readings between twenty-five and thirty-five generally mean you're fine, although the range varies, so that even a reading of forty-five can be considered safe.

Even if your test result is high, cancer may not be the reason. Fibroids can cause high test results, as can endometriosis or even pregnancy. You can get high test results when you're menstruating or recovering from surgery; 1–2 percent of healthy women seem to have naturally occurring higher levels of the tumor marker, causing higher than normal CA-125 results.

A newer test for ovarian cancer called **LPA**, (short for lysophosphatidic acid, a substance that seems to stimulate ovarian tumors), seems to be more accurate for diagnosing ovarian cancer, but still, about 10 percent of the women studied in initial trials had "false positives"—high LPA levels that were either due to a different form of cancer or even due to benign conditions, including fibroids.

If you're getting your first CA-125 (or CA-125II, a new and improved version) or LPA, remember that this is your baseline reading. If the reading seems high to your doctor, more tests, such as a high resolution ultrasound, will be needed to confirm a diagnosis; a more definitive analysis can be done after a biopsy. Even though these procedures are time-consuming and potentially invasive, they can help detect a real malignancy—or more likely, put your mind at ease that your fibroids are benign.

Doppler scan

A cancerous growth sucks blood toward it at a faster than normal rate— even faster, as a rule, than fibroids. A **Doppler scan** (technically, **transvaginal Doppler velocimetry**) can measure how fast the blood in your uterine artery and related blood vessels is flowing toward your fibroids. This could be another step to determine the possibility of cancer. According to the *American Journal of Preventive Medicine*, "Doppler imaging, in combination with transvaginal ultrasonography, improves specificity and ability to discriminate benign and malignant tumors."

The test is generally performed by a radiologist. Much of the procedure is similar to a sonogram: the doctor will cover a probe with a latex covering (similar to a condom), lubricate it, and insert the probe into your vagina. Again, unless you're very dry inside, or very nervous, it shouldn't hurt at all. The doctor will manipulate the probe; my radiologist flipped a switch so that I could actually hear the sound of my own blood rushing through my veins.

Like a sonogram, the radiologist can tell you the results right away; your gynecologist will explain the meaning of the results and put them in context.

Biopsies

A biopsy is a small tissue sample taken from your body and analyzed under a microscope. Your doctor may do a biopsy to check for possible cancer cells, especially if a sonogram shows abnormal growth.

If your fibroids are in the uterine lining, an **endometrial biopsy** can be done to check for cancerous cells. The endometrium, you'll recall, is the lining of the uterus; it can be reached by instruments inserted into your vagina. Your doctor will insert a flexible tube, which has a plunger on one end, into your uterus . The doctor applies a little pressure to remove a sample of tissue from the lining of your uterus.

According to the *Harvard Women's Health Watch*, an "endometrial biopsy is 90 percent accurate in identifying abnormal endometrial tissue"; when it's done in addition to a sonogram, which helps to identify the correct place to get the sample tissue, accuracy goes up to almost 100 percent.

An endometrial biopsy can also be performed using hysteroscopy. The hysteroscope can provide a view of the entire uterine lining, including any areas that show signs of unusual growth.

If your doctor is concerned about fibroids in the wall or on the outside of your uterus, getting a biopsy requires laparoscopic surgery, a procedure that requires checking into a hospital for outpatient surgery. (For more information on hysteroscopy and laparoscopy, see Month 6.)

Gene Identification

A STILL-EXPERIMENTAL genetic test uses reverse transcriptase-polymerase chain reaction (RT-PCR), to identify a specific gene—called the gamma-smooth isoactin gene —that indicates whether a tumor is malignant or benign. If the gene is found in samples taken from uterine biopsies, the tumor is benign. Researchers working on the test consider it definitive—leaving no "grey zone" of uncertainty about whether a tumor is cancerous or not.

D&C

D&C, short for **Dilation and Curettage**, is another procedure used to check for cancerous cells in your uterine lining; it is also sometimes used to try to control very heavy bleeding. Like an endometrial biopsy, a D&C can help your doctor identify malignant cells in the uterine cavity, but it can't test growths in the uterine wall or on the outer wall of your uterus. While an endometrial biopsy samples targeted sections of your uterine lining, a D&C takes cells from the entire lining.

Although a D&C doesn't take very long, it has to be done in the hospital using either local or general anesthesia. It's generally an outpatient procedure. If your doctor detects any problems during the D&C, she may want to explore further by doing a laparoscopy. (See the section on laparoscopy in Month 6.)

The first step of a D&C is dilation to widen the cervix and open the entrance to your uterus. Most often, your doctor will insert a series of small rods, each one slightly larger than the next, to expand the cervix. A more natural (and somewhat slower) alternative is a product called **Laminaria Tents**. These are small tubes, about the size and shape of a cigarette, made from Japanese seaweed; inserted into your cervix, the seaweed absorbs moisture from your body and eventually widens your cervix.

Step two, curettage, comes from the word **curette**, the name of the small spoon your doctor inserts into your dilated cervix and uses to scrape the lining of the uterus.

After having a D&C, you may have cramps, light bleeding, fatigue, or discomfort that can last anywhere from a few days to a couple of weeks. Since your cervix and uterus will be irritated for a while, you should let them rest for three or four weeks after the procedure. This means using sanitary pads instead of tampons, and avoiding intercourse (or any sex play that involves inserting anything into your vagina).

Complications from D&Cs can occur in up to 3 percent of patients; the risks include infection, injury to the cervix, and puncturing the uterus. For this reason, many doctors prefer more technologically advanced techniques, such as hysteroscopy.

Since these new technologies are less invasive, take less time, and—because most don't involve a hospital stay—are less expensive, ask your doctor if there are any alternatives to having a D&C. Bear in mind, D&Cs have been the standard for a number of years; it may simply be the technique with which your doctor is most comfortable.

IN A SENTENCE:

> *Fibroids don't usually turn into—or even mask—uterine cancer, but proper check-ups can put your mind at rest and early detection can be a lifesaver.*

MONTH 8

living

Considering Surgical Treatments

A TEAM of researchers at Duke University, in conjunction with the Agency for Healthcare Research and Quality (AHRQ), conducted an in-depth scientific review of the available literature on fibroid treatments. They created a detailed report, published in the spring of 2001, on the methods available for treating fibroids, and "the effectiveness of their implementation."

The results were discouraging. The report states that, "In general, there was a remarkable lack of high quality evidence supporting the effectiveness of most interventions for symptomatic fibroids." The report goes on to state, however, that "Lack of evidence is not equivalent to evidence of no benefit or of harm. It is possible that some of these interventions are effective in at least some patients. However, the current state of the literature does not permit definitive conclusions about benefit or harm."

So if a team of highly skilled doctors and researchers at one of the top medical facilities in the country couldn't figure out the most effective treatments for women with fibroids, how will you decide what's best for you?

At this point, you've considered the pros and cons of noninvasive treatments such as diet, acupuncture, or even drugs.

Making decisions about more invasive treatment can be stressful, lonely, and complex. Apart from familiarizing yourself with the technical aspects of the different surgical techniques available, the pros, cons, side effects, and benefits, you might experience some emotional reactions. You may find yourself thinking about a changing body image. You may come up against challenges to your feelings of self-esteem, self-confidence, sexual identity. You may need to explore your feelings about having more children—or any children.

Traditionally, many doctors recommend hysterectomy as the preferred treatment for fibroids. As we'll discuss more in Month 11, this is not always because hysterectomies are medically necessary, but because women don't know that alternatives exist.

Women who are informed about their treatment choices, have supportive families or friends, are willing to stand up for themselves, and are able to find a doctor who listens and can share their goals are more likely to choose the treatment that works best for them.

The importance of education. The fact that you're reading about fibroids and their treatments means that you're already doing one of the most important things you can before making a decision about whether to have surgical treatment, and if so, which one is best for you.

The importance of information and support when it comes to making a treatment decision about fibroids can't be underestimated. In Denmark, women with less education, fewer friends, and a less supportive family had double the rate of hysterectomies than their more educated neighbors or those who had stronger relationships with family and/or friends. In Switzerland, a public education campaign in one canton, or state, resulted in a sharp drop in hysterectomies compared to the rest of the country. And in the United States, the more educated a woman is, the less likely she is to have a hysterectomy.

This is not to suggest that hysterectomy is the wrong decision for every woman, simply that a woman benefits from knowing her options.

Getting support. Sometimes, you have to swim against the tide to fight prevailing cultural attitudes. This is a situation where you'll need to call on the most supportive, caring members of your Fibroid Support Team to help you keep focused on what you want and need, rather than what "everyone" seems to be doing.

For instance, doctors in the United States seem to have a stronger preference for recommending hysterectomy than do physicians elsewhere in the world. Women in the United States have more hysterectomies than women in any other Western country, twice as many as women in Great Britain, and four times as many as women in France. And if you live in the South or the Midwest of the United States, you are more likely to have a hysterectomy than women in other parts of the country.

Women of color also seem to get a disproportionately high number of hysterectomies: a Maryland study of more than 53,000 women confirmed that African-American women were 25 percent more likely to have a hysterectomy than their white counterparts. They were also more likely to have surgical complications and a longer hospitalization. Worse, the African-American women in the study were more than three times as likely to die in the hospital, suggesting a range of important questions about quality of care.

There is a tendency for women who've had a particular treatment to recommend it over the other options. Remember, what worked well for your best friend, cousin, or neighbor may have been fine for her—but you owe it to yourself to make your own informed decision.

IN A SENTENCE:

Being educated about all your treatment options and having a supportive network of friends and/or family will help ensure that you choose the treatment that works best for you.

learning

Making Sense of Surgery

IT'S EASY to get confused about your surgical options. There are different types of surgery, different results from surgery, and different tools that doctors can use.

Types of surgery

At its most basic, surgery is either image-guided or direct. Image-guided surgery allows your doctor to perform surgery with a small or no incision, using X-rays (UAEs), or MRI imaging (cryomyolysis), or microcameras (laparoscopy) to guide their movements inside you. Image-guided surgery is used to

- neutralize fibroids inside your uterus.
- remove fibroids and repair your uterus.
- remove fibroids, as well as your uterus and/or ovaries.

Direct surgery is the old-fashioned, but effective, method of opening your abdomen so that your doctor can have the clearest field of vision inside your pelvic cavity. Direct surgery is used to

○ remove fibroids and repair your uterus.

○ remove fibroids, as well as your uterus and/or ovaries.

The choice of which of these two basic techniques is best for you comes down to the size and location of your fibroids, your comfort level with the benefits and risks of each type of procedure, and the skills and recommendation of your doctor.

The following chart shows all the different types of image-guided and direct surgery.

Type of procedure	Fibroids are "neutralized" and left in your body	Fibroids are removed, uterus is repaired	Fibroids and uterus and/or ovaries are removed
Image-guided	UAE	Hysteroscopic resection, a/k/a vaginal myomectomy	Vaginal myomectomy
	Myolysis	Laparoscopic myomectomy	Laparoscopically assisted vaginal hysterectomy (LAVH)
	Cryomyolysis/ I-MRI-guided cryosurgery		Laparascopic hysterectomy
Direct view		Abdominal myomectomy	Abdominal hysterectomy

Results of surgery

Each type of surgery has a different outcome. Here are some criteria you can use to evaluate your treatment decisions, then go to Months 9, 10 and 11 to read about UAE, myomectomy, and hysterectomy in more detail.

IF YOU WANT TO KEEP YOUR UTERUS, EVEN IF YOU'RE NOT INTERESTED IN GETTING PREGNANT
- Neutralizing, image-guided treatments, which shrink or kill off fibroids without physically removing them, include Uterine Artery Embolization, myolysis, cryomyolysis, and I-MRI-guided cryosurgery.*
- Myomectomy, which cuts out fibroids but keeps your uterus intact.

Note: Some of these options, especially UAE, may also preserve your option to get pregnant; we'll look at this issue in Month 9.

IF YOU WANT TO MAINTAIN YOUR OPTION TO GET PREGNANT
- Myomectomy

TO BEST MAINTAIN SEXUAL SATISFACTION
- Image-guided treatments
- Myomectomy
- Supracervical hysterectomy, which removes just the top part of your uterus, leaving your cervix, ovaries, and Fallopian tubes.

IF YOU WERE TO LOSE YOUR UTERUS, BUT WANT TO AVOID GOING ON HRT
- Supracervical hysterectomy
- Total hysterectomy, which removes your uterus, including the cervix, but leaves your ovaries and Fallopian tubes in place.

IF YOU ARE CONCERNED ABOUT UTERINE OR OVARIAN CANCER IN YOUR FUTURE
- Total abdominal hysterectomy, removing your uterus along with the cervix, ovaries, and Fallopian tubes.

Surgical tools

There are four primary tools doctors currently use to perform fibroid surgery. Each type of tool uses a different mechanism for making incisions in your skin, and removing fibroids from your uterus:

○ Traditional instruments, made of cold, hard steel
○ **Cautery** uses electricity to create heat
○ **Harmonic scalpels** use high frequency sound waves
○ **Lasers** use high frequency beams of concentrated light

Many women wonder which surgical tool is the "best" for fibroid surgery. Depending on the skill of the surgeon, each tool can have a varying degree of precision and reduction of bleeding. But there's a difference between the tools used to perform fibroid surgery and the techniques of surgery itself. For instance, "laser surgery" is not a specific treatment: lasers are simply one of many tools a doctor can use to perform surgery. Lasers can be used in myolysis, myomectomy, or hysterectomy; they can be used in abdominal surgery with a large incision or in laparoscopic surgery with a tiny incision.

It's important to consider your doctor's experience and preference for the tools he or she uses. An inexperienced doctor using a laser is a far worse bet than an experienced doctor who prefers cautery or the other tools at his or her disposal.

IN A SENTENCE:

> *Surgical terms can be confusing; the most important thing you need to know are what effects each type of surgery will have on your body.*

Preparing for Surgery

IF YOU choose to have surgical treatment, you can plan on one or more days in the hospital, and usually two to four weeks at home, recovering. Some effects, such as fatigue or abdominal pain, can linger for weeks or months after you go back to work and resume your other normal activities. No matter which treatment you choose, there are quite a few practical things you can do to make your surgery and recovery easier. Your Fibroid Support Team (see Day 4) also plays a critical role.

Prepare your body and mind

Just as you would prepare for a vacation hiking in the mountains, or running a 5K race, you can prep your body for surgery. The three primary ingredients? Exercise, diet, and a positive attitude.

Even if you're not into exercise on a regular basis, you can strengthen your body to recover more quickly from surgery. These four steps can help you focus on important areas to get in shape. (If you're starting to exercise for the first time, check with your doctor.) The sooner you can start an exercise routine before surgery, the more benefits you will get.

○ Strengthen your cardiovascular system with aerobic exercise for thirty minutes, 5–6 times a week. You can try biking, running, speed walking, dance, or other activities that keep your heart rate elevated.

○ Develop stronger stomach muscles with abdominal exercises, such as stomach crunches. Try working up to 100 every day.

○ Your legs and lower back will have to compensate for a weaker abdomen after surgery. Weight bearing exercises will strengthen those parts of the body.

○ Stronger arms will help you accomplish routine tasks more easily after surgery.

Diet, too, plays a part. Healthy, fresh foods will help strengthen your system to respond to the assault of surgery. Reducing sugar, fat, and alcohol (as well as tobacco and any other substances) will free up resources in your body for better and quicker healing. Your doctor may recommend taking the daily recommended amount of iron and folic acid; you can also take a daily multivitamin.

You should stop taking any herbs 2–3 weeks before surgery. Eight common herbs (see box) pose known risks for patients going into surgery, and others may have risks that are yet unstudied. Check with your doctor about any prescription or non-prescription medicine you are taking.

> **EIGHT COMMON** herbs have been found to increase your risk for one or more of the following during surgery: excessive bleeding, irregular heartbeat, lowered blood sugar, exaggerated effects of anesthesia, slow healing or infection of wounds. The herbs are garlic, ginko, ginseng, ephedra, kava, valerian, St. John's wort, and echinacea. Be sure to discuss these or other herbs you are taking with your doctor well before surgery.

Perhaps most important is a good attitude. Meditation and prayer can be powerful tools for releasing your fears and anxieties about surgery. Depending on your comfort level, faith tradition, and desire, you can say prayers for your health and happiness or ask for guidance in facing this challenge and for strength to get through it. Do this as often as you need to; you don't have to wait to be in services at church or in the lotus position in front of your shrine.

Don Cohen, a New York City psychotherapist who prepared six weeks for his own surgery, suggests that this is a particularly rich time to get in touch with your innermost thoughts and feelings. Cohen suggests short-term psychotherapy to deal with anxiety and fear of the unknown as well as more personal explorations: recording and examining your dreams, writing personal healing statements, and engaging in some form of creative expression, like painting or singing.

Cohen extended his mental preparations all the way into the operating room. Instead of being wheeled in to the operating theater, Cohen walked in, introduced himself to the staff, asked their names and requested that they treat him with the same respect and care that they would if he were awake. He also arranged for a nurse to read his healing statements out loud during surgery.

You can try visualizing yourself after treatment as healthy, energized, and free from symptoms. I worked hard at visualizing a perfect outcome for my surgery, although not because I believed I could "create" the future. It was for a more mundane reason: it occurred to me that worrying about problems in advance was a huge waste of energy, and if for some reason the procedure didn't go well, I would have plenty of time to worry about it then. In the meantime, when I woke up in the middle of the night from anxiety, I soothed myself by saying that everything would be fine. (And in fact, it was.)

You can also help relax your body with a massage, gentle yoga, or stretching. Breathing exercises—breathing deeply from your abdomen—can help relieve your anxiety and calm your thoughts.

Last but not least, with all the homework you're doing, you know that whatever you choose to do, you're making a well-informed decision. You can be proud that you've put yourself in charge of taking care of your health.

Prepare your home

Once you get home, you'll need plenty of quiet time and sleep, so organizing your home and responsibilities in advance can make everyone's life easier—especially yours. On a practical level, you won't be able to do any real cleaning for a while, so you may want to give your home a good cleaning before your hospital stay. You can also think ahead about the kind of atmosphere in which you'd like to recover. Depending on how your home is set up, you may want to create a little "recovery nest," including your couch or bed, a low table for food and drink, and easy access to a phone, books, and the TV remote.

I knew that I wanted to come home from the hospital to a clean and restful home, so the night before my surgery, I spent some serious time cleaning and straightening up (it was also a good use of all my anxiety-fueled energy). I did the laundry and arranged my apartment so that I could come home to a freshly made bed, clean towels, and a sparkling bathroom and kitchen. If you like, this is a good opportunity to ask someone from your Fibroid Support Team to help you out.

Pre-surgery shopping

Shopping for several weeks' worth of nonperishable foods (cereal, canned goods, bottled juices, and so on) can ensure that your family can make do while you're recovering. If you're the person who prepares the family meals, cooking and freezing meals in advance can also relieve you of those duties to some extent when you come back from the hospital (and keep your loved ones fed while you're gone). Of course, cooking meals before or after surgery is another good task to delegate to a member of your Fibroid Support Team.

The week before surgery, I stocked up on a few things I would need in the first few days after I came home. I bought canned soup, Jell-O®, crackers, and other things that could keep. I also stocked up on cranberry juice to help ward off a possible urinary infection after surgery.

The other shopping stops I made pre-surgery were:

- ○ the drugstore, to make sure I had the things I usually run out of, like toothpaste, deodorant, and toilet paper; plus ibuprofen for possible post-surgery pain and sanitary pads for post-surgery bleeding (a little is normal);
- ○ the bookstore, where I got a few titles that I'd always wanted to read (and now would have four weeks at home to indulge);
- ○ the bank, where I took out enough cash to see me through a few weeks of food and grocery deliveries;
- ○ the health food store, where I got arnica gel and Bach's Rescue Remedy Creme®, both highly recommended by friends for reducing the appearance of scars; a bottle of acidopholous capsules, to

help normalize my intestinal activity after surgery, and a box of Emer'gen-C™, a powder that, mixed with water, promises an "energy boost" and provides healing antioxidants.

Arranging child care and/or pet care

If you've got kids, or even pets, depending on you, don't assume that you can take care of them alone when you get out of the hospital. Well before your hospital stay, think about your options for support. If you have a spouse or partner, talk honestly about how much time he or she can devote to child care and/or pet care and then see what you need to do to fill in the gap. Certainly, if you're the only adult in the house, you need to arrange for some help.

If you have children living with you, find time to talk with them about what's happening. Depending on how old they are, they may have questions that need your reassuring answers. At a minimum, you'll need someone to look after them for about a week. Prepare your kids as if you were leaving town for a few days. Write out lists to help keep them (and their caregivers) organized, buy and cook supplies of foods they like to eat, and perhaps even leave a few little love notes or gifts that they can find while you're in the hospital.

For pets, perhaps there is someone in the neighborhood who can walk your dogs or look in on your cats, feed them, and give them some reassuring pats. If your finances permit, look into boarding your pets with a local vet for a week or so. Your pre-surgery shopping list should include plenty of pet food and other necessities.

After you're home, it will be hard for you to be up and running right away, so if you can, consider extending your caregiving arrangements for an extra week or so.

Preparing at work

This can be a tricky area. While many employers are understanding and flexible, others are more concerned with getting work done than about your health. As a rule, I would suggest telling people at work about your health on a "need to know" basis, putting professionalism first.

Quietly check your company policies before approaching your boss about taking time off for surgery. Knowing what the company has put in writing will help you keep discussions focused on what the company allows and then making a case for any personal exceptions you require.

Before I confided in my boss or co-workers that I needed surgery, I took the following steps:

○ checked my company's short-term disability policy to determine my rights on the job;
○ checked with the company's human resource manager to see how much sick time/vacation I was still entitled to for the year (in addition to short-term disability time);
○ evaluated my work load to determine which projects would need to be covered while I was out.

Since there is rarely a "good" time to take off from work, I scheduled my surgery according to my own and my doctor's timetable. Two weeks before the surgery was to happen, I notified my boss. I told him, briefly, that I needed surgery and that it was important. I was able to tell him the official company policy on short-term disability, how much time I was entitled to take off, and how I suggested covering my work responsibilities while I was gone. Fortunately, my boss was very understanding. I was able to take off four weeks and return to my job.

You might feel comfortable sharing details about your medical condition with your co-workers, but you certainly are not obligated to do so. You might have the kind of relationship with your boss that allows you to negotiate the best time to schedule your operation, but again, the decision is not contingent on your boss's priorities.

If you work for a company of more than fifty people, or a public school, you may be protected under the Family and Medical Leave Act. If you're not covered by the FMLA, you still may be covered by state laws; you can check your rights with your State Attorney General, Equal Opportunity Employment Commission, or State Department of Labor.

Preparing your friends/support group

Everyone I know has a different idea about who they want to see while they're in the hospital and while they're recovering at home. One friend preferred almost total isolation, except for her husband, until she was up and walking again. Another went to her home state to have surgery so she could recover in the home of her father and stepmother. Personally, I wanted to have a party in my hospital room, though once I got home I preferred having only one visitor per day. Whatever you want, you're free to arrange; again, it's a question of your priorities.

E-mail is a great tool for letting people know what you want. A friend who preferred no hospital visitors sent out a lovely note explaining her condition and asking for prayers on the day and hour of her surgery. (If you belong to a religious community, such as a church, mosque, or synagogue, you can request prayers from the congregation you belong to as well.) I sent an e-mail out to my friends and family, detailing when I would be in the hospital, the hospital address and phone, and how long I expected to be there. I invited everyone on the list to come visit me in my hospital room, and happily, many did.

More specifically, you can ask people from your Support Team to help you with particular needs. I tapped my oldest friend to be my health care proxy, the person who could make health care decisions on my behalf if I became incapacitated. I arranged for someone to go to the hospital with me on the morning of my surgery. Your friends will no doubt have their own creative ideas: for instance, a few people stopped by the hospital while I was in the operating room to sit with and comfort my parents, who had come from out of state.

Whether you choose to be with family or friends, consider arranging to have someone with you in the hospital for the first day and evening after surgery. It's nice to have someone there if you need to reach your glasses or a tissue; even in the best hospital, nurses are not available every moment to give you water, help you to and from bed, or hold your hand.

I was enormously gratified and touched by the response of the people I know: having surgery turned out to be a wonderful way to find out how much I am loved. It started by my speaking up and saying I needed help. I hope that your experience is as rewarding in terms of getting the right kinds of support from your friends and family.

Packing for your hospital stay

If you have UAE or laparoscopy (belly-button surgery), you will probably stay in the hospital one night; if you have more extensive surgery (abdominal myomectomy or hysterectomy) you will probably stay three to four nights. Your doctor will be able to give you a reasonable estimate. So the night before surgery, you'll need to pack a little bag for your stay in the hospital.

The first rule, of course, is not to take anything too valuable. While you're in surgery, everything you've brought to the hospital will be in a locker; later, in your hospital room, there will be numerous people going in and out and unfortunately many opportunities for things to go missing. So jewelry, credit cards, and so on are best left at home. You'll need a small amount of cash for things like renting a TV in your hospital room; if you can, ask a friend or relative to bring this to you after you're out of the recovery room and in your hospital room. Finally, make sure your overnight bag is labeled clearly with your name; I used an old canvas duffel that I could write my name on with black marker.

The second rule is to take washable items. After a stay in the hospital, it's a good feeling to be able to throw everything you've used into the washing machine to clean away any stray dirt, germs, and those strange hospital smells. Even my canvas bag was machine washable.

After arriving at the hospital on the morning of surgery, I was led to a locker room where I changed from my own clothing into cotton hospital pajamas. I did wear those hospital-issued jammies for the duration of my four-day stay, but I also had a cotton kimono that I brought for extra coverage, and a large pink fake Pashmina shawl for warmth and color. (When my doctor came to see me the day after surgery, she exclaimed that I was the most stylish patient there.) Since my feet are often cold, I also brought a pair of slippers.

For going home, you'll need clothes that are not binding, especially around the waist; a loose dress is perfect. Since you'll need to use sanitary pads for a few days after surgery, you will need to wear underwear: big old-fashioned bloomers (or something close) are better than tight little bikinis, since you don't want binding elastic anywhere close to your incision. I also found it easier not to deal with a bra for the short trip home from the hospital. Since bending over can be painful, shoes that you can just slip on, with no laces, buckles, or zippers, will be easiest; flat, rubber-soled shoes will help you walk more securely.

In addition to the normal personal care items that you always travel with, such as toothbrush and toothpaste, you might want to consider including the following:

Informed Consent

BEFORE YOUR treatment, your doctor should let you know the circumstances that would change your procedure during surgery. For instance, a laparoscopic procedure (with a small incision) may need to become a laparotomy (a large incision) if the surgeon finds more problems than anticipated. If you have specific instructions, put them in writing for your doctor and the hospital; it could also be helpful to have a family member or good friend available during surgery who can confer with your doctor on your behalf, if necessary. You will be given a form to sign. You can amend this by hand if you have specific wishes, such as avoiding hysterectomy unless your life is in danger. Be sure to discuss your instructions with your doctor and make sure he or she supports your wishes.

○ cough drops for the little coughs that can develop after surgery (coughing with an incision is not fun);

○ a prepaid phone card or a phone credit card number for long distance calls;

○ light reading (I found that Harry Potter was great company in the hospital!);

○ a personal stereo with headphones (this is one of those items that you might want someone to bring you after you're in your hospital room);

○ if you normally wear contact lenses, you will not be able to wear them during surgery. Consider leaving the contacts at home and wearing your glasses for the duration of your hospital stay.

IN A SENTENCE:

You can do a lot to ensure your hospital stay and recovery are as easy as possible.

learning

Considering Uterine Artery Embolization (UAE)

UTERINE ARTERY Embolization (UAE) is a technique used since the late 1970s to stop hemorrhaging after childbirth and pelvic surgeries. In 1995, it was used for the first time to reduce the size and symptoms of fibroids. (For that reason, it is now sometimes also called UFE, for Uterine Fibroid Emboliza-tion.) More than 5,000 women in the United States, and 15,000 worldwide, have had UAE to reduce their fibroids and fibroid symptoms.

UAE is done in a hospital setting by a specialist called an Interventional Radiologist (IR). Strictly speaking, UAE is not surgery, since nothing is cut from your body, and your fibroids are not removed. Still, it's an invasive procedure with its own set of risks and benefits.

When you have UAE, tiny particles are injected into your uterine arteries, which drastically cut down the flow of blood to your fibroids. When the blood supply is cut off, the fibroids shrink, and in some cases, die. If you remember our discussion of degeneration on Day 1, you'll remember that sometimes this happens naturally. UAE, in effect, makes all your fibroids degenerate at the same time.

Specifically, UAE has been shown to be effective at controlling troubling symptoms:

- ○ stopping or improving vaginal bleeding and chronic pelvic pain in 70 to 96 percent of women, depending on the study.
- ○ reducing feelings of pressure in anywhere from 61 to 96 percent of women.

Some fibroids may be better candidates for UAE than others; sessile fibroids in the lining and uterine wall (submucosal and intramural) appear to shrink the most. Fibroids growing closer to the outer wall of the uterus (subserosal), and pedunculated fibroids, those on a stalk, are less likely to be affected.

UAES TAKE surgical procedures, and income, away from gynecologists. If your gynecologist doesn't recommend UAE, ask why—and then do your own homework. In the best case, your IR and ob-gyn will work together both to ensure your safety and evaluate your results. In addition, some insurance companies, though not all, have denied coverage, saying that UAE is experimental; your IR may be able to help you deal with this.

WHO IS THE "BEST" CANDIDATE FOR UAE?

While UAE is technically available to any woman with fibroids, doctors identify the ideal candidate as someone who . . . .

- ○ doesn't want (more) children, or is willing to take a 1 to 2 percent risk of infertility;
- ○ has significant symptoms caused by fibroids;
- ○ is being told that she needs a hysterectomy and doesn't want one;
- ○ has no history of prior pelvic irradiation or **renal failure**;
- ○ has had an ultrasound and/or endometrial biopsy, with no evidence of malignancy, chronic infection, or alternative explanations for symptoms;

○ has sessile (ball-shaped) fibroids that are submucous (in the lining) and/or intramural (in the wall).

UAE MAY ALSO BE A GOOD CHOICE FOR SOMEONE WHO . . . .

○ wants to avoid the possibility of blood transfusions for health or religious reasons;

○ is not able to have general anesthesia;

○ wants to keep her uterus intact and has been told by her obstetrician/gynecologist that a myomectomy will probably not be successful.

YOUR RISK WITH UAE MAY BE HIGHER THAN AVERAGE IF:

○ you're taking certain medications: for example, synthetic progesterone, found in some birth control pills and other medications, can contribute to UAE failure;

○ you have endometriosis (presence of the endometrium in abnormal places), chronic salpingitis (inflamed Fallopian tubes) or **endometritis** (inflamed endometrium), which increase your risk of infection;

○ you've ever had pelvic irradiation or **vascular disease**;

○ you've already had surgery for fibroids, which may make UAE less successful;

○ your fibroids are very large. Although there is no fixed size limitation for UAE, Dr. Jacques Ravina, the first doctor to perform UAE for fibroids, reports that women with very large fibroids may still need to have them removed surgically after UAE, since large submucous fibroids can become infected or cause uterine prolapse and large subserous fibroids can form adhesions, leading to bowel obstruction.

YOU ARE NOT A CANDIDATE FOR UAE IF:

○ you have any kind of active infection, especially a pelvic infection;

○ you're pregnant;

○ you've been diagnosed with a gynecological cancer;

○ you have an allergy to contrast dyes (although if you're aware of the allergy, appropriate medication before the procedure can make it safer);

○ you have had renal failure;

○ a biopsy or ultrasound reveals a source of bleeding unrelated to fibroids;

○ your fibroids are pedunculated subserosal fibroids (hanging in the uterine cavity) or cervical fibroids (fibroids growing on the cervix).

Having UAE

Before scheduling your UAE, you'll need to have a Pap smear and a sonogram or MRI (see Day 2 and Month 6 for more information about sonograms and MRIs). This is to make sure that your fibroids are the cause of any symptoms you have and that you don't have any other conditions, such as endometriosis, that could rule out having UAE. If you're bleeding heavily and persistently, you may need an endometrial biopsy to rule out the possibility of cancer (see Month 7 for a description of this procedure). If any other tests are suggested, ask about the risks as well as what the doctor plans to learn.

Once you are approved, and have decided to have the procedure, you'll schedule a hospital appointment. UAE takes about an hour or two to perform, but if you're like most women, you'll need to stay in the hospital for a day or so.

Unlike typical surgery, UAE doesn't require a large incision or general anesthesia; there is virtually no blood loss, and bleeding episodes that require transfusion are rare. UAE is done under conscious sedation, meaning you're tranquilized but awake while the procedure is going on; some doctors also use a local anesthetic, similar to an epidural, to numb you from the waist down.

Once you're sedated, a slender tube called a **catheter** —no wider than a matchstick—is inserted into the large artery near your groin. The puncture mark is about where the elastic on the bottom of your underwear hits your leg. You're injected with a special dye, which can make you feel warm or give you the illusion that you need to urinate; the dye shows up on an X-ray machine, which the doctor uses to guide his movements. (A newer variation uses MRI instead of X-rays, which can increase the precision of your doctor's view.)

When the catheter is in your uterine artery, the doctor releases tiny particles, no larger than grains of salt, called **PVA (polyvinyl alcohol)**. Then, since most of us have two uterine arteries, the catheter is guided to the other artery and additional PVA is released.

The flow of your blood directs the particles to small blood vessels in the walls of your uterus, where they lodge and slow down the flow of blood to your uterus. Reducing the blood flow in your uterine arteries causes your fibroids to degenerate. Remarkably, the normal tissue in your uterus isn't harmed, as the main uterine artery is not touched by the PVA particles.

After the procedure, you'll lie down for at least six hours, while the IR monitors you for any complications or drug reactions. During this time, most women have cramps or pelvic pain, which typically last anywhere from six to twelve hours. The IR will give you pain relief, which can range from NSAIDs (such as ibuprofen) for mild pain to an intravenous morphine pump.

While some women feel well enough to be discharged from the hospital the same day, most stay overnight for pain management. By the follow-

> **AS AN** alternative to PVA, your doctor may use a substance called gelfoam. While PVA stays in your body indefinitely, gelfoam is temporary, dissolving in your body ten to twenty days after the procedure. Doctors are examining whether a one-time insertion of gelfoam could be enough to shrink fibroids and relieve symptoms. In addition, clinical trials are being held for a new type of material to block the uterine arteries, called embosphere microspheres. The advantage of the microspheres are that they should be easier to inject and target; microspheres have already been approved for use in Europe, Australia, and Canada.

ing morning, any pain you feel should have improved, though it won't go away entirely for a week or two. You should get a prescription for pain relief before you leave the hospital. (The size of your fibroids has nothing to do with how much pain you may experience, and pain is not an indication of whether the procedure worked or not.) You may have a bruise where the catheter was inserted. A pink or brown discharge is also common for a few weeks or even months after the procedure; this is the remnant of degenerating fibroids.

The normal recovery time is fairly short. Most women are able to get back to their normal activities in four to ten days. The results of UAE might be immediate, or could take weeks. As far as how much fibroids will shrink, reports are mixed, but overall, UAE has reduced fibroid size anywhere from 29 percent (about one-third) to 88 percent within three months of the procedure; the average reduction is in the range of 50 to 67 percent. If the UAE works, fibroids can continue to shrink for up to twelve months, but experts caution that if there has been no change after six months, the UAE was not effective. Your IR should examine you, using ultrasound or MRI, at four to six weeks after the procedure and again at three, six, and twelve months.

Most women to date are very satisfied with the result of their UAEs. At the 16th World Congress of the International Federation of Gynecology and Obstetrics (FIGO), doctors reported that 80 to 90 percent of women undergoing UAE had "significant improvement" in heavy bleeding, feelings of pain or pressure, or both, and as a result, saw big improvements in their quality of life. Follow-up studies done at six months and one year after the procedure showed that the effects of the procedure had lasted at least that long.

The longest follow-up done to date—over the course of six years—showed no recurrence of fibroids. A different study, after two years of follow-up, found new fibroids in two women (3.5 percent of the fifty-eight women in the study). Since other studies are underway, you might want to ask this question again if you start to investigate the procedure for yourself.

Risks

Compared to myomectomy and hysterectomy, UAE is relatively new. As a result, the long term effects of UAE are unknown, but we do know of some side effects that merit your consideration.

After UAE, some women develop a temporary condition called post-embolization syndrome. This usually feels like a fever, but can resemble menopause, complete with hot flashes, mood swings, and cramping that can last anywhere from a few days to as long as six weeks.

Other symptoms, including fever, chills, discharge, and pelvic pain, can mean you have an infection. If you have any of these problems, make an appointment with your gynecologist; antibiotics can usually clear up a pelvic infection. If the symptoms are very severe, including nausea, vomiting, and abdominal pain, you may have to check back in the hospital for a brief stay.

In addition, there are some potentially serious side effects of UAE:

○ **Misembolization** happens to 1 to 2 percent of women having UAE. If particles from the UAE get into the wrong place, they can damage other pelvic organs—most notably your ovaries. If your ovaries are embolized, they stop functioning, which means that you will go into menopause. One review of the literature suggests that for women over forty-five, the risk of misembolization and ovarian failure may be as high as 15 percent.

○ **Fibroid slough**, spontaneous discharge of your fibroids through the vagina, is a possible side effect that can occur between two and seven months after the procedure. Usually, the fibroids are passed without incident, but if expelling them is painful, you may have an infection. If this happens, talk to your IR or gynecologist immediately; you'll need antibiotics to cure the infection, and possibly a procedure like a D&C (see Month 7) to remove any remnants of the fibroids that are still in your uterine cavity. The average risk of fibroid slough in two studies was about 3 percent.

○ **Injury to the uterus.** About 1 percent of women have an injury to the uterus—infection or blood loss—that's severe enough to require a hysterectomy.

○ **Lack of symptom relief.** Approximately 10 to 15 percent of women do not find enough symptom relief from UAE; many of these women go on to have either a myomectomy or hysterectomy. Studies show that 5 to 10 percent of women who had UAEs later had a hysterectomy, possibly signifying an unspecified problem, or a return of fibroid symptoms.

○ **Mortality.** So far, UAE has proven to be very low-risk for the most serious complication of all. As of this writing, only two deaths have been reported out of approximately 15,000 procedures performed worldwide. In comparison, reported rates of deaths from hysterectomies are one in 1,000 (that is, fifteen deaths in every 15,000 operations).

Sex after UAE

Many of the sensations of sex and orgasm come from the blood that fills the uterus and vagina when you're aroused (see Month 3). Since sex is a subject many women—and their doctors—find difficult to discuss, the effect of UAE on arousal and sexual sensation is not yet clear, although recent, preliminary studies give us an indication of the possibilities.

A survey conducted by Georgetown University among 115 women who'd undergone UAE found that the procedure did not have a negative effect on the women's sex lives, and in a few cases, may have improved them. A small survey at Yale found that 43 percent of post-UAE patients had more interest in sex than they had before the procedure, and 27 percent reported stronger orgasms.

However, there are several ways in which UAE could create problems with your sex life. The most serious possibility is misembolization of "non-target" blood vessels in and around the uterus, which some doctors report, "may interfere with some patients' sexual response."

UAE may have a negative impact on sexual feelings in two other ways. The first is how it might affect the ability of the uterus to fill with blood. In some women, the very mechanism that makes UAE effective in shrinking fibroids—that is, slowing the flow of blood in the uterine arteries—may prevent the uterus from filling as fully with blood when you're aroused; this would affect all the sexual sensations following from that. Women used to having uterine orgasms before UAE have expressed some concern that after the flow in the uterine arteries was slowed down, their orgasms aren't the same as before. For women who had serious symptoms, especially heavy bleeding, the trade-off was necessary . . . but it's still a trade-off.

There is also a possibility that UAE may damage the nerves going into the uterus. It's easy to forget, but nerves are living tissue and need blood to function properly. Blocking the blood supply to the nerves going into the uterus may damage those nerves. If you were used to feeling pleasureable sensations in your uterus, you may no longer feel them after the embolization.

Remember, these are only possible side effects, and not all women experience uterine orgasms. Some sources suggest that the sensation is only felt, or noticed, by about a third of all women. If you're in that third, take note, and be sure to have a strong heart-to-heart with your doctor before the procedure.

Pregnancy after UAE

As we saw earlier, one of the issues about UAE is how often it may affect the ovaries, and whether this effect is confined to women over forty (although this is young enough for many women to still consider motherhood). So far, all the reported cases of ovarian failure have been in women over forty years of age, and most over forty-five.

Although there are women who have had successful pregnancies after having had UAE, the effect of UAE on fertility has not been well-studied. However, the possibility of ovarian failure is one reason IRs are very cautious about recommending UAE to women who are still interested in having children.

For this reason, doctors agree that myomectomy is still the standard of care for women with fibroids who both need medical treatment and hope to maintain their fertility. This is not to say that myomectomy will ultimately prove better than UAE, only that it has a known track record.

IN A SENTENCE:

> UAE shrinks fibroids by starving them permanently of blood; it has helped thousands of women get relief from their fibroids, but there are potential complications which you should weigh carefully before choosing this treatment.

Myolysis and Cryomyolysis

THESE ARE two related techniques that, like UAE, kill off your fibroids while leaving them inside the uterus. **Myolysis**, also known as **myoma coagulation**, uses heat to kill the fibroid and its blood supply; **cryomyolysis** uses extreme cold.

Myolysis was first used for fibroids in 1984, but its use has been limited. Recently, doctors have started to improve the precision of targeting fibroids using Magnetic Resonance Imaging (MRI); these advances may make the techniques more widely used.

New studies show that MRI technology, guiding laser light directly to your fibroids, shrinks fibroids by about a third. (This technique is also called "**percutaneous laser ablation**.") While this is less shrinkage than you might get with UAE, the procedure is apparently less painful and women are able to leave the hospital within about six hours after surgery.

The surgery is performed with laparoscopy, following one to three months of GnRH agonist therapy. During surgery, the doctor inserts four thin, hollow needles into your abdomen, guiding them to the fibroids with MRI. Special laser-conducting fibers are then inserted through the needles into the fibroid, where they are heated to over 140 degrees, killing the fibroid cells. The fibroid continues to shrink for about six months. (In cryomyolysis, a similar procedure, fibroids are targeted and killed by probes that are cooled to less than 360 degrees below 0 F.)

Myolysis and cryomyolysis are both possible treatments for women who aren't planning to have children. There are some women who've conceived after these procedures against their doctors' advice, running the risk of uterine rupture. It's possible that the greater precision afforded by MRI may one day make this technique safe for women who want to maintain the option to get pregnant. However, until the risks have been fully explored, you might want to pass on both myolysis and cryomyolysis if you want to conceive in the future.

MONTH **10**

living

Considering Myomectomy

MYOMECTOMY IS surgery in which your doctor removes your fibroids, and leaves the rest of the uterus intact, or repairs the uterus to be (almost) as good as new. Although the surgery is less destructive than hysterectomy, only one myomectomy is performed in this country for every five hysterectomies done for fibroids. According to the National Center for Health Statistics, only 35,000–40,000 myomectomies are performed in the United States each year.

Although a myomectomy can be major surgery, there are considerable advantages over hysterectomy: once you recover, you maintain sexual feelings, bladder control, and hormone production. You maintain your ability to create a child, if that is important to you; you retain all of your reproductive organs, keeping you whole both physically, and in some cases, emotionally.

Keep in mind that you can have a myomectomy at any age, no matter how many children you have or are planning to have. You can have a myomectomy even if you are not planning to have any more children or any children at all. You are entitled to keep your uterus, no matter what (barring cancer). Only in extreme cases are your fibroids too large for an experienced surgeon to remove.

After considering my own options carefully over five years, and after researching and writing my first book on fibroids, I opted to have a myomectomy. I'd been told many, many times since my early thirties that I needed a hysterectomy, or as I got older that I "might as well" have one. A **DES daughter**, I'd had an ovary removed at age seventeen; it has been an article of faith for me that I didn't want to lose another organ. In addition, I don't have children, and didn't want to lose the option of having them. And despite numerous incidents of **cervical dysplasia** (cells mutating in the cervix), I didn't want to take any drastic measures to prevent a cancer I might never get.

When I finally did have a myomectomy, after five years of "watchful waiting," it was because sonograms had revealed that my fibroids were growing fast. There were three fibroids visible on the sonograms: The largest one seemed to fill up the whole back of the uterine cavity. Over the course of three months, that particular fibroid seemed to quadruple in size. I had only the most minor symptoms: occasional pain and pressure, a feeling of fullness; I never had irregular bleeding, cramps, or other problems. But the growth was a signal to me that I had to do something.

My decision to have a myomectomy was based on what seemed best for me. I evaluated my options, and my feelings about them, and decided I was most comfortable with surgery that didn't leave a residue in my body, as UAE does. (The decision I made is not the only possibility; it was simply right for me. I have spoken to many women who opted for UAE over myomectomy and they are also very happy with their choice. Other treatment options currently being tested will provide a wider range of options in the near future.)

The day of the myo, not surprisingly, was stressful. It helped that a friend picked me up at home early in the morning and rode down to the hospital with me. I filled out my insurance and financial information; I wrote down the names, addresses, and phone numbers for my next of kin and health care advocate—the person who would speak for me if I could not. My advocate was one of my oldest friends, whom I'd briefed extensively on my wishes for treatment—and if absolutely necessary, what I wanted in terms of extreme lifesaving measures.

I also had to fill out a consent form, which outlined what I was allowing my physician to do in the operating room. I trusted my doctor; I like her enormously. We had talked many, many times about my need to keep my uterus. But if I signed the form as it was written, I would be giving my permission for the doctor to do whatever she thought necessary. I fished in my bag for a pen and amended the form by hand: I did not give permission to remove my uterus under any circumstance. Extreme as it might sound, I preferred to be closed up, woken up after surgery, and go back the next day if I had cancer or any other life-threatening problem.

Later, lying in the waiting room to be prepped, I made the same point to the interns who came to prep me for surgery, and to my doctor when she came to escort me to the operating room. The one condition I consented to was on the unlikely chance that I was bleeding to death; in that case, I grudgingly agreed that my doctor could perform a hysterectomy.

The surgery was a **laparotomy**, that is, open abdominal surgery. This was partly because the fibroids had become too large for most doctors to do a laparoscopic surgery and partly because I was most comfortable with my doctor having a completely clear field of vision to find all the fibroids and repair my uterus as needed. I knew I would have a large incision; it was about eight inches long, and ran horizontally just above the bikini line. Per my doctor's instructions, in the weeks before surgery I donated two units of my own blood (one unit, or pint, per visit); my doctor also used a cell-saver to recycle my blood during surgery. In the event, I lost about 20 percent of my blood volume, but did not need a transfusion.

Anesthesia in the past has left me feeling nauseous for weeks; when I asked the anesthesiologist about this, he was able to give me Zofran®, which worked beautifully to prevent post-op nausea. In the operating room, the anesthesiologist smiled kindly at me and told me to count backward. I woke up in the recovery room. The surgery had taken four hours; it had been a success. The fibroids were gone and my uterus was intact.

Later I found out that the fibroid we'd seen on the sonogram had filled my entire uterine cavity: the intern smiled and cheerfully told me they'd had to "core me like an apple." Pathology showed that while the fibroids were benign, the cells were mutating—a possible precursor to cancer. Instead of the three fibroids that had shown up on the sonogram, I had twelve: six large, three medium, and three small.

I stayed in the hospital four days. Pain relief was a little bit of a problem in the hospital; despite my doctor's intervention, I did not get pain medication as often as I felt I needed it. Day three was particularly hard as the pain medicine from surgery wore off.

On day four, I was discharged, and once again, a friend saw that I got home. I was moving slowly and stiffly, but I managed to walk a couple of blocks to buy some fruit. Then I came home and collapsed on the couch.

I stayed home for about a month. I slept a lot. I read all four Harry Potter books. I felt able to have one visitor a day; the rest of the time I kept the phone turned off, but left a message on my answering machine to let my friends know I was all right and would call them back when I woke up. Even though I live alone, I was able to do everything I needed: turn on the shower, turn on the stove, go to the grocery. I didn't lift anything heavy for several weeks; my doctor had told me not to try to pick up anything heavier than five pounds.

By two weeks I was feeling normal enough to go out for lunch in the neighborhood, and take walks longer than around the block. At four weeks, I went back to work, but limited my other activities so I could get plenty of rest. At eight weeks, I still noticed small twinges and some fatigue; this lasted until the fourth month. At that point, I felt a new infusion of energy; I was myself again.

IN A SENTENCE:

> *Having a myomectomy was not the only choice, but it was the best choice for me.*

learning

Types of Myomectomies

MYOMECTOMY OPERATIONS can be done one of three ways:

- ○ vaginally, on an outpatient basis
- ○ using laparoscopy, also on an outpatient basis but with a longer recovery period, or
- ○ through abdominal surgery.

The kind of myomectomy that could be best for you depends on the number, size, and location of your fibroids, your surgeon's experience and skill, and your preferences. Of course, you need to find a doctor comfortable with and skilled in myomectomy. Bear in mind, that even with the best of intentions, a myomectomy may turn into a hysterectomy in the operating room because of medical need.

IF YOU'RE planning to have a myomectomy or hysterectomy, you may want to consider donating two pints of your own blood in case of possible blood loss: this is called an **autologous donation.**

Vaginal myomectomies

Most often called **hysteroscopic resection**, this procedure can only be done if you have relatively small fibroids inside the cavity of your uterus. It's most effective for pedunculated fibroids, the kind that grow on a stalk inside your uterus. These are also the fibroids most likely to cause symptoms of heavy menstrual bleeding or to prevent conception. Doctors studying resection in the Netherlands say it is best if you have no more than two fibroids, although women with more fibroids may also benefit.

The way it works is this: Using the hysteroscope, as we saw in Month 6, your doctor will insert a miniature camera inside your vagina; your uterus will be filled with saline solution to expand the walls. Then, using another tool, your doctor will shave your fibroids away bit by bit, until they're at the same level as the wall of the uterus.

Resection won't work if you have fibroids anywhere but the uterine cavity or the uterine lining. This is because only the part of your fibroid that is inside the cavity of your uterus can be shaved away; anything inside the wall or on the outer wall will still be there, siphoning blood and interrupting the normal working of your uterus.

There are various tools your doctor can use for hysteroscopic resection, including a laser, a cutting electrode, or a vaporizer. Most of the time the procedure is done without making any cuts in either your skin or inside your uterus, but some doctors prefer inserting a laparoscope in a tiny incision near your belly button; this improves their vision inside the uterus and can help prevent the risk of perforation.

Some doctors will recommend that you take a GnRH agonist for a month or two before surgery to shrink the fibroids or to reduce the possibility of bleeding (see Month 4 for more on GnRH agonists). This is because a smaller uterus helps make the surgery easier and safer; the reduced blood flow to the uterus leads to less blood loss during surgery and less need for a possible transfusion. If your doctor recommends taking GnRH agonists, consider the benefits and risks of these drugs before beginning treatment—and consider the possibility of surgery that uses a larger incision, without drug treatment.

The surgery takes about thirty minutes and can be done on an outpatient basis, but it's safer to have a hysteroscopic resection in a hospital that has the latest fluid management equipment. Fluid overload is one of the most frequent—and most dangerous—risks of hysteroscopic resection. The problem is that your body can absorb the saline solution that's pumped into your uterus during surgery. Make absolutely sure that your doctor will be using a machine with an automated fluid management system, which not only measures fluid going in and coming out, but sets off an alarm if your fluid intake is too high; Dr. David Olive of Yale University Medical School advises that you "should insist upon it" for your surgery.

Only about 10 percent of ob-gyn physicians actually perform resections; another 20 percent have been trained but don't perform the procedure because even they lack the necessary expertise. Your doctor should have advanced certification from the ACGE (the Accreditation Council for Gynecologic Endoscopy) in order to perform hysteroscopy.

Endometrial Ablation?

ENDOMETRIAL ABLATION can help stop abnormal uterine bleeding (AUB), one of the top reasons, after fibroids, that women get hysterectomies. Ablation works by burning or even freezing the inside of the uterine lining (the endometrium), where new blood vessels grow every month before menopause. After having endometrial ablation, you're technically able to conceive, but probably unable to have a baby, so it's not appropriate if you still want children–though you'll still have to use birth control to avoid a tubal pregnancy.

But if fibroids are the reason that you're bleeding, ablation alone won't help. While ablation destroys the lining of the uterus, it doesn't affect any fibroids you may have. Experts, including the FDA, agree that you should not have endometrial ablation if you have fibroids.

Laparoscopic myomectomy

Laparoscopy is minimally invasive surgery; it can be used to perform a wide variety of surgeries, among them, myolysis, cryomyolysis, myomectomy, and hysterectomy, including supracervical hysterectomy.

In Month 6 we talked about a "test" laparoscopy, where a mini camera is lowered into your abdomen. The difference in a surgical procedure is that in addition to the camera, the doctor makes one or more small cuts lower down on your belly, near the bikini line; each of these cuts might be no larger than the size of a short fingernail. The doctors use these tiny incisions to insert a wide variety of instruments that can cut, grasp, remove, or repair.

The camera sends images of your insides to a video monitor; the surgeon and operating room staff move the instruments while they watch what's happening on the monitor.

The doctor will remove the fibroids in very small pieces, generally with the help of a mechanical device called a **morcellator** (which chops your fibroids up into small "morsels" and suctions them out of your body). If your fibroids are too large to remove laparoscopically, your doctor might elect to perform what's called a " laparoscopically assisted" procedure. In this case, the cut near your bikini line might have to be enlarged to several inches.

Depending on the size and number of your fibroids, of course, the operation generally takes about two hours; in one study of 368 women, fewer than 3 percent needed a blood transfusion (for which the women had donated their own blood).

One of the most common side effects of laparoscopic surgery is urinary tract injuries; this happens to 10 percent of the women who have laparoscopic myomectomy. It can take as long as three to four months to recover from these injuries, and you might need additional surgery. The skill and experience of the surgeon is critical to minimize potential problems in this area.

Other potential complications from laparoscopy include:

○ damage to the intestines.
○ nicked blood vessels.
○ damage to the bladder or kidney tubes.
○ damage or scarring of the gynecologic organs, which may create fertility problems in the future.

While laparoscopies can be done on an outpatient basis, most doctors will keep you for a twenty-three-hour "day," so you can be observed in the hospital overnight. (Some physicians offer "office laparoscopy," but this is not recommended, as you'll receive more complete care in a hospital or fully equipped outpatient surgical center.) One to two weeks after going home, many women feel ready to go back to work.

Again, your doctor may recommend that you take a GnRH agonist, especially if your uterus is very large or you've become anemic (see Month 4 for a discussion of GnRH). As we said in the previous section, if your doctor recommends taking GnRH agonists, consider the benefits and risks before beginning treatment.

Abdominal myomectomy

There are several reasons you and your doctor might opt for abdominal surgery for your myomectomy:

○ your fibroids are large and/or numerous;
○ laparoscopic surgery would take much longer, requiring you to be under anesthesia for more time;
○ your doctor has significant experience with this technique;
○ abdominal surgery allows the surgeon the greatest field of vision, an important consideration for removing fibroids and other growths that may not have appeared on an ultrasound;
○ it's easier for the surgeon to make sure all blood vessels have been tied off and the surgery is "clean" before he or she is finished;
○ if you are planning to get pregnant, some doctors believe that abdominal myomectomy allows the surgeon to close the incisions most securely.

Before the operation (sometimes just minutes before), you'll talk to the anesthesiologist. This is your chance to discuss any allergies you have; in particular, if you know that anesthesia makes you nauseous, the anesthesiologist can give you a drug to counter this effect.

Once you're in the operating room and under anesthesia, your pubic area will be shaved, and your doctor will make a six- to eight-inch horizontal incision, most often just above the pubic bone, at your bikini line. A vertical cut may be necessary if your uterus is quite large (often more than "twenty-four weeks" in size).

During the operation, your surgeon will elevate your uterus to see the fibroids as clearly as possible; he or she will remove them with one of a number of tools, including a scalpel (knife), laser (light), or cautery (heat).

The method is less important than your surgeon's skill, comfort, and experience with his technique.

Before you can go home after surgery, you need to be walking, eating, passing gas, urinating, and not have a fever; this can take anywhere from two to five days. Once you go home, the recovery period can vary, from two to six weeks, but even if you go back to work sooner, plan on taking care of yourself with extra rest, lots of fluids, and light, healthy foods.

INTERNAL SCARRING, *or adhesions,* are one of the leading causes of post-surgical complications, from both abdominal and laparoscopic surgeries. After any kind of surgery, internal tissues can join together (adhere to each other), which causes scar tissue to form. Adhesions can form from tissues being touched or simply exposed to the air.

Adhesions generally form within the first few days following surgery. While they normally don't cause problems, they're associated with up to 20 percent of infertility cases and are found in up to half of the women who have chronic pelvic pain after surgery. A type of plastic film is available that may help keep adhesions from forming; ask your doctor about the possibility of using this or a similar product if you need surgery.

Risks

Myomectomies, like all surgeries, come with a set of risks. In addition, there are several considerations that may affect your decision to have this surgery:

Blood transfusion. During surgery, 10 to 15 percent of women having myomectomies need transfusions, compared to 5 to 10 percent of women having hysterectomies. The risks associated with having a transfusion are far less if you use your own blood (making an autologous donation two or more weeks before surgery), or if your doctor uses a cell-saver to recycle your blood during the operation.

Lack of symptom relief. After surgery, about 20 percent of women still have problem symptoms, which could indicate that fibroids were not the original source of the problem. The "cure" rate for myomectomy, based on relief of symptoms, is about 80 percent—meaning four out of five women see their conditions improve.

Uterine scarring. Myomectomies can scar your uterus, which would lower your chances of getting pregnant. This is why many doctors will suggest you try to get pregnant before seeing if you need surgery. However, if you can't conceive or maintain a pregnancy, and fibroids are the reason why, a myomectomy will often improve your chances. Uterine scarring is also called **Asherman's Syndrome.**

Your fibroids may return. This is the most common argument used against having a myomectomy. Over the course of time, there is a 10 to 20 percent chance—some say up to a 30 percent chance—that your fibroids will grow back or that new fibroids will develop. However, there is a greater chance—70 to 90 percent—that they will not. Even when fibroids grow back, you often get a five- to ten-year "window" of relief from symptoms. And any new fibroids may not give you any problems at all. Studies show that 8 to 10 percent of women having myomectomies went on to have hysterectomies for recurrent fibroids.

Sex after myomectomy

If you remember our discussion of uterine contractions in Month 3, we talked about how fibroids can prevent those contractions. Quite simply, myomectomy, in removing the fibroids, removes the problem. Once a woman has a myomectomy, the contractions resume.

If you've been in pain, had heavy bleeding, or other serious symptoms, myomectomy, like the other procedures available, can improve life dramatically. Myomectomy preserves your anatomy in a functional way, and for the women who find this important, maintains their body image as a complete, whole, and healthy woman.

Pregnancy after myomectomy

While there are no guarantees, about two-thirds of the women who want to conceive after myomectomy are able to. But once you've conceived, miscarriage is still a possibility. Estimates of delivery rates—successful pregnancies—after myomectomy range anywhere from 40 to 80 percent.

As we mentioned earlier, some doctors feel that the **sutures**—the stitches or staples used to repair your uterus—used in laparoscopic myomectomy may not be as secure as in a regular myomectomy. If you decide you want laparoscopic surgery before trying to conceive, you'll need to find a very skilled, very experienced surgeon with specialized training who can perform the complicated suturing technique to repair your uterus firmly enough to carry children. If your fibroids are in the wall of your uterus (intramural), even the most experienced surgeon may not be able to repair your uterus so that it's strong enough to carry a child; in this case, you might want to consider choosing an abdominal myomectomy.

Once you've had abdominal surgery, such as a myomectomy, the internal scars (adhesions) can sometimes cause infertility. If this becomes a significant problem for you, a skilled doctor can clean up some of the adhesions laparoscopically or through hysteroscopy (vaginally).

Myomectomy also creates a small risk for **uterine rupture** during pregnancy. Your risk for uterine rupture after myomectomy is in direct proportion to how many incisions your doctor had to make in your uterus to remove your fibroids; if you had an extensive myomectomy, your doctor may recommend delivery by C-section to avoid the possibility of rupture.

As we saw earlier, fibroids can reappear after a myomectomy. But not everyone gets new fibroids after a myomectomy, and even if you do, they may not interfere with your chances of conceiving. There's usually a window of opportunity to become pregnant after you recover from surgery and before any new fibroids have a chance to grow large enough to affect you.

Having said all that, it probably is helpful to time a pregnancy as soon after surgery as you're ready. If you wait too long, and if your fibroids do come back, larger ones may interfere with your ability to carry your baby to term without complications.

IN A SENTENCE:

> *Myomectomy is a proven surgical technique that removes your fibroids and preserves your uterus.*

living

Considering Hysterectomy

SHOULD YOU have a hysterectomy? It is a good answer for many women who want a permanent solution to their fibroid symptoms and have thought through their other options, as well as their reaction to losing their uterus and possibly their ovaries. The key issue here is that, most of the time, having a hysterectomy is up to you. (See Month 8 for tips on making a decision about medical treatments.)

A hysterectomy is permanent. That could be good news or bad news: if you never want to have your period again, worry about getting pregnant, or be concerned about having fibroids or any other uterine condition, hysterectomy can provide you with those things (though, as we'll see later, not without a certain amount of risk). On the other hand, if you change your mind about wanting your uterus back, for physical or psychological reasons, you can't undo the surgery.

More than 600,000 hysterectomies are performed each year in the United States; about one third to one-half of these are for fibroids. (This figure is provided by the CDC, which also reveals that the number should be higher, since the agency doesn't track vaginal hysterectomies, hysterectomies done in VA hospitals, and other categories.) According to a study by the

THE FIRST recorded hysterectomy was done in the 2nd century c.e., by the Greek gynecologist, obstetrician, and pediatrician, Soranus of Ephesus.

RAND Corporation, the societal costs of hysterectomy include $1–2 billion in hospital and related expenses each year, plus up to 7 million days of lost productivity. Collectively, women getting hysterectomies spend over 900,000 days per year in hospitals, which is more hospital time than recorded for patients with AIDS, breast cancer, or prostate cancer.

By the time a woman in the United States reaches age sixty, there is a one in three chance she will have had a hysterectomy; compare that to the United Kingdom, where the rate, while arguably still high, is one in five. Surprisingly, most hysterectomies in the United States are performed on women who are in their reproductive years.

○ Between 1988–1993, 55 percent of all hysterectomies were done on women aged thirty-five to forty-nine years; the majority of these were done on women under forty.
○ A look at the records of almost 1,800 women showed that the average age of hysterectomy was 42.5 years.
○ Of the 60 million women of child-bearing age in the United States, 3 million (as of 1995) have had a hysterectomy: that equals one woman in every twenty.

Doctors agree that in cases of cancer, a hysterectomy is mandatory: this accounts for 10 percent of the hysterectomies done in this country every year. (A little-known surgery called radicaltrachelectomy can preserve the uterus in some cases of early-stage cervical cancer, although a hysterectomy is still considered absolutely necessary for cancer affecting the body of the uterus.) Hysterectomies are done for women when their lives are at stake because of emergency bleeding or complications during pregnancy; there are also plenty of women who've researched their options and feel that hysterectomy is the choice they prefer. But that leaves a very large number of hysterectomies for fibroids which may be unnecessary:

○ A Blue Cross/Blue Shield study found that 30 percent of hysterectomies were unnecessary, as they were "performed for fibroids and other benign (noncancerous) conditions."

○ *U.S. News and World Report*, after reviewing data from insurers in seventeen states, stated that "as many as 1 out of 3 hysterectomies is medically unnecessary."

○ Researchers at the University of California, looking at the medical records of 500 women, found that 70 percent had hysterectomies for inappropriate reasons, including doing inadequate workups before surgery and not exploring less invasive treatments first.

○ An editorial in the *British Medical Journal* notes that among premenopausal women, 70 percent of hysterectomies are done for "perceived abnormal bleeding," when the menstrual blood loss is really within the "normal" range.

The problem with hysterectomy is not that it exists or is used as an option for women who have fibroids. The problem is that many, many doctors will recommend a hysterectomy and not tell you about your other options.

A survey on behalf of the Society for Women's Health Research shows that two-thirds of American women don't know that they have alternatives to hysterectomy for treating excessive menstrual bleeding, let alone other conditions, including fibroids. The same survey showed that doctors recommend hysterectomies to one in four women. Of those women, 82 percent accepted their doctors' recommendation. In many cases, women who had a hysterectomy did not even discuss potential alternatives with their doctors.

In many cases, doing your own research, as you're doing right now, is the only way to tell whether a hysterectomy is really the right choice for you. NBC Medical Correspondent Dr. Bruce Hensel wrote that "No woman should submit to a hysterectomy without considering all the options." The article was entitled "Hysterectomy Should Be Last Resort."

Perhaps you're considering a hysterectomy to take care of your fibroids or fibroid symptoms, but still aren't sure it's the right answer for you. Assuming that your doctor hasn't given you a diagnosis of cancer, how many of these other conditions apply to you?

○ You have chronic severe pain and/or heavy menstrual bleeding due to one or more large fibroids.

○ You do not want to have any (more) children.

○ You've tried gentle, natural alternatives for your symptoms.

○ You've explored the surgical options which preserve your uterus (UAE, myomectomy, and others) with your doctor or even better, a specialist who does one or more of these procedures routinely.

○ You have had one or more routine tests to confirm your doctor's diagnosis, such as an endometrial biopsy or a presurgical laparoscopy.

○ You're comfortable with the idea of your sexual and feminine identity with or without your uterus.

○ You've gotten a second, third, even fourth opinion. (Fortunately, since hysterectomies are considered elective surgery, most insurance companies will pay for a second opinion.)

If you said "No" to all, or even most of these points, you may want to go back and reconsider some of your other options. However, if you said "Yes," you are prepared to look at hysterectomy as a viable alternative.

IN A SENTENCE:

> *Consider your options—and your feelings about them—before deciding to have a hysterectomy.*

learning

Types of Hysterectomy

THERE ARE three basic types of hysterectomy: the key difference is in how much of your reproductive system is removed:

○ part of the uterus (**supracervical**, also called subtotal or partial hysterectomy)

○ the entire uterus (**total hysterectomy**, also called simple hysterectomy, partial hysterectomy, or complete hysterectomy)

○ the entire uterus, plus ovaries and Fallopian tubes, **total abdominal hysterectomy** (**TAH**), also called **hysterectomy** [or total hysterectomy] with bilateral **salpingo-oophorectomy**, **hysterectomy** with bilateral **oophorectomy**)

Supracervical hysterectomy

Supracervical hysterectomy (also called subtotal or partial hysterectomy), leaves you more intact than any other type of hysterectomy; your doctor takes out only the back of your uterus, leaving the cervix attached; you also keep your ovaries and Fallopian tubes. The big advantages are that your bladder and bowel function, and your sexual response, are preserved better than in any other hysterectomy. You may also have less risk of surgical and postoperative pain and complications.

The first successful supracervical hysterectomy was performed in Manchester, England, in 1843. Until the 1950s, it was the hysterectomy of choice for many women and their doctors. But it began to seem dangerous when cervical cancer was discovered as a major killer, and most doctors began performing total hysterectomies—taking out the entire uterus, including the cervix. Now, however, as we saw in Month 7, an annual Pap smear can detect cervical cancer with a high degree of accuracy, and many gynecologists and patients worldwide have questioned the routine removal of the benign cervix.

The surgery for a supracervical hysterectomy is most often done using laparoscopy, or microsurgery. Going through a small incision near your belly-button, the surgeon cuts the back of the uterus (the "balloon" part) into small pieces and suctions them out. The cervix is left attached to the muscles in your pelvis. This means that your cervix continues to anchor these muscles, as well as your vagina; the shape of the vagina is not changed, as it is in hysterectomies which remove the cervix.

You will be able to have this operation unless you have prolapse of the cervix, cervical dysplasia, or cancer. Experts say that women can have this surgery with fibroids up to a sixteen-week size, sometimes even a little bigger.

Total or radical hysterectomy

If you and your doctor have a conversation about hysterectomy, be sure to clarify the language he or she uses very carefully. A "total" hysterectomy means taking out your entire uterus, including the cervix. You keep both ovaries and Fallopian tubes. However, in a "total abdominal hysterectomy," all of your reproductive organs are removed: the uterus, cervix, both ovaries, and Fallopian tubes. More extreme, a "radical hysterectomy" also includes removing the supporting ligaments, tissues, the upper portion of the vagina, and in case of cancer, the pelvic lymph nodes.

Each type of hysterectomy can be performed vaginally, laparoscopically, or abdominally; the method usually depends on the size and/or number of your fibroids. Some of the surgical issues and side effects particular to each type of operation are discussed in the individual sections which follow. Afterwards, we'll review the overall risks associated with hysterectomy.

Your Ovaries

IT IS extremely important to know that removing your ovaries is not necessary when you have surgery for fibroids. On the contrary, there's a very strong argument for keeping them.

The ovaries produce estrogen, as well as progesterone and small amounts of testosterone. (See Week 2 for the effects of these hormones.) After menopause, your ovaries don't "die," but still produce tiny amounts of these hormones, continuing their beneficial effect to a small degree. If you opt for surgery that removes both ovaries (known as a "bilateral oopherectomy"), you will enter what is called surgical menopause; this is both more sudden and often more severe than natural menopause.

If you're considering hysterectomy of any kind, it's important to know that the ovaries may need the uterus to continue to function: injury to arteries during surgery may cut off their blood supply, causing them to stop working. About a third of the time, ovaries left in place after hysterectomy stop functioning.

Still, in a study of almost 700 women, those who kept their ovaries were much more satisfied with their hysterectomies than those who didn't. One important reason is sex: how much you want sex, how often you have it, and how easily you achieve orgasm all seem to be easier when you have your ovaries.

For women willing and able to take Hormone Replacement Therapy (HRT) after their ovaries are removed, it's important to know that these drugs don't bring your hormone levels back to where they were before surgery. Dr. Stanley West, in his book *The Hysterectomy Hoax,* is emphatic: "There is no substitute for natural hormones . . . You need your ovaries."

The surgical terms that refer to your ovaries are:

○ "Salpingectomy," surgery removing one or both of your Fallopian tubes;

○ "Oophorectomy," surgery removing one or both of your ovaries;

○ Since these procedures are almost always done together, the combined procedure is called a "Salpingo-Oophorectomy."

Vaginal hysterectomy

Most vaginal hysterectomies are done for fibroids smaller than a twelve- to fourteen-week size, though some doctors have been able to remove fibroids as large as twenty weeks. The operation is literally done by taking your uterus out through your vagina, with no external incision.

The benefits of having a vaginal hysterectomy are that the operation itself tends to be shorter (though it can last over two hours, depending on the difficulty of the operation), leave no visible scar, and probably no internal scarring. Since you don't have to heal from an incision, your recovery time should be quicker than it would be for abdominal surgery.

On the other hand, since your doctor isn't able to see inside your entire abdominal cavity, there is greater potential to damage the bladder and rectum. A less serious risk is urinary tract infection, which can affect up to half of the women who've had a vaginal hysterectomy.

One thing to be aware of is that vaginal hysterectomies are so easy—for your doctor—that some may be tempted to suggest it as a quick and simple solution for your fibroids. Dr. Herbert Goldfarb, in his book *The No-Hysterectomy Option: Your Body—Your Choice*, warns against vaginal surgery which is too quick and seems too easy: "The 'thirty-minute' vaginal hysterectomies that doctors boast of performing are often procedures that don't have to be done in the first place!"

Laparoscopically Assisted Vaginal Hysterectomy

If your fibroids are too large for a vaginal hysterectomy, your gynecologist may recommend a **laparoscopically assisted vaginal hysterectomy(LAVH)**, which adds the element of laparoscopy to a vaginal procedure. If it's appropriate, LAVH can be much easier on your body and promote a quicker recovery than traditional abdominal surgery. But remember, LAVH becomes technically impossible if your fibroids are too big.

The average time for LAVH is about an hour and a half; the hospital stay is usually two to three days, though some women go home the day following surgery.

The complications for LAVH include damage to the urinary tract (1–2 percent) and hemorrhage requiring transfusion (3–4 percent). In one study,

5 percent of the operations had to be converted into an abdominal hysterectomy.

LAVH can, in seemingly many cases, help convert a possible abdominal hysterectomy into an easier procedure. However, it's still more invasive than a regular vaginal hysterectomy, if that is indeed an option for you.

Abdominal surgery

As we saw in Month 10, many doctors prefer performing abdominal surgery for both hysterectomies and myomectomies. Abdominal hysterectomy is the simplest of all the surgeries you could be offered, and is standard training for all gynecologists.

Like an abdominal myomectomy, an abdominal hysterectomy takes place in a hospital: it requires general anesthetic and an incision that is usually six to eight inches long. Unlike a myomectomy, however, the surgery is usually only about half an hour. This is because, instead of carefully removing your fibroids and repairing the uterus, the surgeon ties off the arteries and ligaments connecting the uterus to the rest of the body, cuts them, and simply lifts the uterus out of the pelvis.

Your hospital stay will usually last for three to five days; total recovery generally takes four to six weeks. See Month 10 for more details on how to prepare for your hospital stay, surgery, and recovery.

Risks

Removing your uterus can create a number of problems. Of course, pointing out a risk doesn't mean it's definitely going to happen. If you're satisfied that the benefits of having a hysterectomy outweigh the risks, and it feels like the right decision, you're more likely to be happy with the outcome.

There are three sets of risks: those associated with the operation itself, side effects that may show up shortly after the operation, and longer-term complications.

The immediate risks of the operation itself include:

○   perforated vagina
○   bladder or ureter injury

O bowel injury
O intestinal scarring
O infection
O blood clots
O blood loss requiring transfusion

As is true with any surgery involving general anesthesia, the effects of the drugs may linger, making you feel moody, tired, or weak for a few days after surgery.

It is important to note that doctors consider hysterectomy a safe procedure. However, up to 50 percent of women have minor complications, such as a urinary tract or pelvic infection. The rate for major complications, such as bowel injury or blood clots, is 1–2 percent; the death rate is 0.1 percent. This means that for the reported 600,000+ hysterectomies performed each year in the U.S., there are an estimated 6,000–12,000 serious injuries, and approximately 600 deaths.

Shortly after hysterectomy, you may experience one or more of the following:

Surgical menopause. As we discussed earlier, surgical menopause is the result of losing both ovaries. Since you lose the protective effect of the hormones the ovaries produce, surgical menopause is both more sudden and often more severe than natural menopause. According to the National Center for Health Statistics, women lose both ovaries in almost half of all hysterectomies; in a study tracking women between thirty-five and forty-nine years old, over half (56 percent) lost their ovaries. Discuss this issue very carefully with your doctor to be sure you agree on what will be removed during your hysterectomy, and what will not. Again, removing your ovaries is not necessary when you have surgery for fibroids.

Self-image. Some women experience separation from their uterus as a blessing, a relief, or even as a practical matter. For other women, losing the uterus represents a loss of femininity, or makes them feel incomplete. There's no right and no wrong, only a question of understanding how you feel and accepting what you need. If you must have a hysterectomy and feel that you would miss your uterus, you may need a period of mourning during or even after your recovery from surgery.

Changes in sexual response. After hysterectomy, you may experience a change in how you respond to sex. Some women experience a new freeness, leading to greater desire and enjoyment. Other women lose their libidos, experience pain or dryness, miss the sensations in their uterus during orgasm, or worse, even lose their ability to have an orgasm.

Unless you have a supracervical hysterectomy, a hysterectomy can hurt your sex life through:

○ accidental perforation of the vaginal walls
○ shortening of the vagina, leading to painful and difficult penetration
○ formation of pain-causing scar tissue in the vaginal cuff
○ vaginal dryness

We'll discuss sex after hysterectomy in more detail later in this chapter. (See Month 3 for a complete discussion of the role your uterus plays in sexual satisfaction.)

Depression. Changes in hormones, self-image, and post-surgical problems, if any, all contribute to depression after hysterectomy. Studies suggest you might be more likely to experience depression after a hysterectomy if:

○ you weren't offered any other options for treatment
○ you have a history of depression
○ the surgery isn't essential to treat a life-threatening condition
○ you're unhappy in your marriage or relationship
○ you still want to have children

If you absolutely need or desire a hysterectomy and you think depression might be an issue for you, you can help prepare yourself. For instance, counseling can be a helpful outlet to talk about fears of losing your femininity, not being able to enjoy sex, or even how the operation may affect your spouse or partner. Including your partner in your fears, medical considerations, and decision-making process, talking, or even going to counseling, can increase his or her understanding of what you're going through—and how the two of you can get through this together.

Other possible side effects of hysterectomy include weight gain, chronic pelvic pain caused by internal scar tissue (adhesions), and urinary incontinence (the inability to hold back urine).

In the long term, hysterectomy is seen to be a possible risk factor for heart disease. This may be due to the loss of hormones produced by the ovaries, which are increasingly thought to have a protective effect on the cardiovascular system. In addition, prostaglandins, produced by the uterus, help prevent blood clots from forming in the arteries. Without that protective effect, clotting can increase the risk of cardiovascular disease.

The findings about hysterectomy and heart disease depend on whether women lost their uterus, ovaries, or both:

○ As early as 1981, data from the ongoing Nurses' Health Study, involving more than 120,000 nurses, showed that women under thirty-five, whose ovaries were removed when they had their hysterectomies, were over seven times more likely to have a serious heart attack before age fifty-six than those whose ovaries were left intact.

○ In 1987, the British medical journal *The Lancet* reported that women who'd had a hysterectomy for fibroids had three times the rate of heart disease than women who'd had myomectomies.

○ In 1997, the University of Pittsburgh School of Medicine found that women whose ovaries were removed when they had their hysterectomies had higher levels of blood pressure and "bad" cholesterol than those who'd kept their ovaries.

○ In 2000, in a study of more than 17,000 women, Swedish researchers reported that pre-menopausal women who lost both ovaries increased their risk of heart attack; after natural menopause, hysterectomies of any kind increased a woman's risk of heart attack by 380 percent.

Sex after hysterectomy

Giacomo Berengario da Carpi of Bologna, an Italian physician and surgeon, recorded the first instance of an altered sex life following a hysterectomy . . . around the year 1500. Five hundred years later, the idea of sex being the same, worse, or better after hysterectomy is still being debated.

Surveys show that 50–60 percent of women report that their sex lives are better after hysterectomy, though we don't know how these women would have felt after a less invasive procedure. And a certain number of women experience no change. (Unfortunately, none of the studies distinguish between the different types of hysterectomy, though a supracervical hysterectomy is more likely to keep sexual functioning intact.)

But a fairly large percentage of women feel that their sex lives are seriously hurt, if not destroyed, by hysterectomy. According to *The American Journal of Obstetrics and Gynecology*, 33–46 percent of hysterectomized women have partial or total loss of sexual function, difficulty becoming sexually aroused, or reaching orgasm.

A review of studies shows the disparity in results, but also shows that women whose sex lives are better, worse, or the same after hysterectomy break down roughly into thirds:

Out of every 100 women . . .

Women reporting no major changes in their sex lives:	16–47%
Women who report better sex lives after surgery	34–70%
Women who report that their sex lives got worse	13–46%

Various studies also show how different aspects of sex got better, worse, or showed no change after hysterectomy. (The numbers don't always equal 100 percent, due to inclusion of various study results.)

	% Better	% Worse	% No Change
Frequency of sex	21–56	12–47	–
Interest in sex (libido)	16–23	32–46	30
Of those who had orgasms before	9	17–25	63
Of those who had no orgasms before	65	–	35
Of those who had painful sex before	85	–	15

The unrealistic idea that all women will have a single type of sexual response after hysterectomy, and that it will uniformly be positive, is a notion that many doctors (and even some post-hysterectomy women) cling to. As we've seen, many women do experience good results. But many others do not. If you are considering having a hysterectomy, evaluate your sex life just as carefully as you would any other aspect of your health and well-being, and make sure your doctor shares your concern—and interest in—your having a happy, fulfilling sex life.

IN A SENTENCE:

> *If you decide to have a hysterectomy, you still have options, and risks, to consider.*

MONTH **12**

living

Staying Healthy

YOU'VE DONE it. You've lived with your fibroids for a year and you've taken one of what I imagine will be several steps in getting the most information you can on the topics that interest you most, whether it's improving your lifestyle, reducing stress, deciding to take herbs or prescribed medications, or exploring one of the many types of surgery available.

That's a lot of work.

But as you've already realized, while this book will end, your own story will continue. But you won't be on your own.

Now that you're informed about fibroids and their treatments, you can reach out to help other women you know if they get their own fibroid diagnosis. You can help them understand that they have options and that they can take control of their treatment plans, and their own good health.

In the meantime, let's talk about you some more. As long as you have your fibroids—and even after you decide to treat them, if you do—you can still use this book as a reference. Go back to Day 3 when you need a fresh incentive to keep your Lifestyle and Symptoms Indicator. When you feel like you need the support of a caring friend, or someone to keep you company at the movies, go back to the Fibroid Support Team you first listed on Day 4. Don't underestimate the power of your friendships to tide you over the rough spots . . . and brighten up other occasions.

When you need a refresher on your diet and exercise program—and who doesn't?—take another look at Days 5 and 7, and renew your commitment to a healthier style of living.

If your period starts getting heavier, if you start spotting between periods, if you start experiencing any symptoms at all, or more symptoms, look back to Week 2 for help in keeping a record of what's going on with your body; sharing this information with your health care provider will help him or her give you a better diagnosis.

And of course, there's more. Keep your medical history updated; if you haven't created a medical history yet, go back to Week 4 when you're ready for a sample format. And if any of the other topics become more pertinent later on—from sex to pregnancy, drug therapy to surgery—check back in these pages as often as you need.

New developments are bound to happen. Researchers in both the United States and other parts of the world will discover new answers to what causes fibroids and makes them grow. Doctors, medical researchers, and medical technicians will develop and test new medicines and technologies to improve the treatment of fibroids. And women speaking out will continue to improve the prognosis for everyone who suffers from fibroids.

Stay informed. Stay active in your health care. Be proud of how well you're taking care of yourself . . . and will continue to.

IN A SENTENCE:

While your experiences with fibroids continue, you can still rely on this book and your other resources to see you through.

learning

Staying Informed

AT LAST count, there were 26,000 health-related websites out there. In 2001, according to *Time/ON* Magazine, 41 million people will use some of these sites . . . a number that is projected to double by 2005. But how accurate or trustworthy is the information you find online?

A study by the California Health Care Foundation and the RAND Corporation found that most of the time, health information on the Internet is hard to find, hard to read, and often incorrect or incomplete, even on the best sites. The study showed that government and university sites did better than commercial ones.

Dr. James Metz, editor-in-chief of the nonprofit Oncolink site, was quoted in the *New York Times* as saying "Too many sites are just trying to sell something, and it is scary how they can make a bad site look good."

And Jason Girzadas, a partner in the health care consulting practice of Deloitte Consulting, was quoted about health care websites in the *Wall Street Journal*, saying "The tools out there [on the Internet] are disorganized, and to a large degree not trustworthy."

One study found that websites offered contradictory information on the same site and the same topic 53 percent of the time; even on top-rated sites, researchers found complete and accurate information only 45 percent of the time.

The lesson is, you can find valuable information on the Internet . . . but don't assume any new nugget of information is correct. Double check, triple check, and as much as possible track down the original source of the information.

In order to help sort through the confusion, I've compiled a highly selective list of organizations, books, websites, and e-mail discussion groups which I have found most helpful in my search for information on fibroids; I have no relationship to any of the resources listed here, and nothing to gain by recommending one over another.

Here are a few tips for judging the information you find on these sites, in the books, magazines, and newsletters I've also listed, and in sources you find on your own:

○ Doctors do not consider studies "proven" until they have been done several times by unrelated teams of researchers . . . and all the results are similar. The most reliable studies are those done with two groups: a test group that receives treatment, and a matched "control group," which does not receive treatment.

○ Press releases about the results of new studies sometimes camouflage the fact that an FDA-approved treatment may be years away.

○ The larger and longer-term the study, the more reliable the results. One good example is the Harvard Nurses' Study.

○ Be especially cautious about information that comes from commercial websites or newsletters, even those from doctors or clinics: while the information they offer may be accurate, they are often trying to sell you something. Check any interesting information from these sites with non-profit, government, or university sources.

○ Credible health-related websites, newsletters, and magazines usually have an editorial board or listing of the names and credentials of those responsible for the medical content; ideally, you should be able to contact these professionals by phone, e-mail, or fax with questions.

○ Look for references or links to other sources of information: a reputable resource will not position itself as the only source of information on a topic.

○ Check when a website was last updated; according to the FDA, health and medical websites should be updated weekly or monthly.

○ Your key word is balance: If something sounds too good to be true, it often is. On the other hand, if something sounds like a terrible idea, consider the source. Remember, in online chat rooms and bulletin boards, you don't know if the people posting bad (or good) experiences are representative of all the women who've had a particular treatment.

○ If you come across a website that you suspect is fraudulent, you can check with the FDA by e-mail at otcfraud@cder.fda.gov.

The resources listed, especially those on the web, should allow you ample opportunity to find additional links. The newsletters and magazines recommended also often offer sources for further reading in the articles they publish.

As you know, organizations move, phone numbers change, websites migrate; please be patient if by the time you read this, any contact information provided here is out of date. As you'd expect, these recommendations are meant to be helpful in your continuing search for information about fibroid treatment, but I am not responsible for the content of any of the resources mentioned here.

A Word About Websites

○ For simplicity, all website addresses have been abbreviated. Each address shown should begin with http://. For example, the *New York Times* website, listed here as www.nytimes.com, needs to be input in your computer as http://www.nytimes.com.

○ If you have trouble with long web addresses (those that include lots of slashes) try this: log on to the home page first, then enter the additional information. For instance, to get to the Times section on women (listed below as www.nytimes.com/women), go to http://www.nytimes.com; when you get the main screen, type "/women" after the address to reach the section on women.

○ For websites where I have not listed information beyond the basic address, you can use the site's navigator to search for information on fibroids by typing "fibroids" into the search window and progressing along the links.

Glossary

ABDOMINAL MYOMECTOMY: Surgery that removes your fibroids, performed via an incision in the lower abdomen. Also see myomectomy.

ABDOMINAL SONOGRAM: Type of sonogram in which the probe is run over the outer skin of your belly.

ABDOMINAL SURGERY: Surgery that takes place through an incision that is usually 6–8 inches long, low on the abdomen. Can be used to perform both myomectomies and hysterectomies.

ACUPRESSURE: A Traditional Chinese Medicine (TCM) technique, similar to acupuncture, which uses pressure on key points in the body to promote healing.

ACUPUNCTURE: Part of TCM, acupuncture is a healing technique that uses needles to stimulate Qi at key points on the body.

ADENOMYOSIS: A condition in which parts of the endometrium (the uterine lining) are somehow pushed deeper into the uterine wall. While adenomyosis is not thought to be cancerous, it can cause a lot of pain and abnormal bleeding.

ADHESIONS: Internal scarring caused by internal tissues joining together (adhering to each other). Adhesions are a leading cause of post-surgical complications.

ALTERNATIVE MEDICINE: An inclusive term for a huge variety of treatments not considered standard in Western medicine, including acupuncture, massage therapy, biofeedback, homeopathy, and many other techniques.

AMENORRHEA: Condition in which a premenopausal woman has not had a menstrual period for at least 6 months.

AMNIOTIC FLUID: Protective liquid that surrounds the fetus during pregnancy.

ANABOLIC STEROIDS: Artificial hormones given to many animals raised for food, to make them bigger and heavier, and provide more meat per animal.

ANDROGENS: Primarily male hormones that woman have in small amounts.

ANEMIA: Deficiency of iron (hemoglobin) in the red blood cells. The amount of blood loss in a single day that could start causing anemia is between 2 and 3 ounces, or about a quarter of a cup.

ANGIOGENESIS: The creation of new blood vessels.

ANTIPROGESTERONES: A class of drugs that suppress **progesterone**, the other major hormone, besides **estrogen**, that our **ovaries** produce, and one which recently has come under scrutiny for its role in **fibroids'** growth. (Also called antiprogestins.)

ARACHIDONIC ACID: A substance contained in the fat in dairy products, that stimulates our bodies to produce **prostaglandins**.

ASHERMAN'S SYNDROME: Scarring of the uterine lining.

ASPARTAME: The ingredient in popular sugar substitutes.

AUTOLOGOUS DONATION: A donation of your own blood prior to surgery, for use in case a blood transfusion is needed.

AYUR-VEDA: A healing system thought to have originated 5,000 years ago: called the "mother of all healing" for its influence on Chinese, Greek, Western and holistic medical theory.

BENIGN: Not cancerous.

BETA-ENDORPHINS: Hormones that create relaxing or pleasurable feelings.

BETA-CAROTENES: A natural substance that provides the color in certain vegetables, helps protect the body against **free radicals**, and converts into vitamin A.

BFGF (BASIC FIBROBLAST GROWTH FACTOR): A hormone which helps control the growth of uterine cells.

BGH (BOVINE GROWTH HORMONE): Given to dairy cattle to increase milk production. Unfortunately, BGH produces IGF-1, a hormone that may have a role in fibroid growth, as well as in prostate cancer and breast cancer.

BIOCHEMICAL TUMOR MARKER: Higher levels of this marker in your blood may indicate the presence of cancer cells. Readings between 25 and 35 generally mean you're fine, although the range varies, so that even a reading of 45 can be considered safe.

BIOPSY: A small tissue sample taken from your body and analyzed under a microscope to check for possible cancer cells.

BIRTH CONTROL PILL: A popular form of contraception, also prescribed to reduce bleeding and slow the growth of fibroids.

BLACK COHOSH: An herb used in a popular form of HRT known as RemiFemin®, as well as other brand name preparations.

BLADDER: The organ that stores urine, prior to expelling it.

BMI (BONE MASS INDICATOR): A test that measures bone density.

CA-125: A blood test used to help diagnose ovarian cancer. It is not a "screener" for cancer; high test results can be caused by a number of benign conditions.

CAESAREANS: See C-section.

CANDIDA: A yeast-like infection which can lead to a more serious disease if left untreated.

CARNEOUS (RED) DEGENERATION: The term used for **fibroids** that **degenerate** during pregnancy.

CATHETER: Slender tube used in surgical procedures.

CAUTERY: A surgical instrument that cuts tissue with heat.

CBC (COMPLETE BLOOD COUNT): Comprehensive blood tests, which show, among other things, whether you're anemic.

CERVICAL CANCER: Cancer of the **cervix**, most commonly detected with an annual **Pap smear**.

CERVICAL DYSPLASIA: Cells mutating in the **cervix**.

CERVICAL MYOMA: A rare type of fibroid found on the **cervix**.

CERVIX: The small ring of muscle that forms the opening to the **uterus** and connects it with the **vagina**. The cervix is connected to the pelvic bones and ligaments, which help keep our pelvic organs in place.

CHAKRAS: An energy system defined by Hindu philosophers in India thousands of years ago. Seven chakras ascend from your groin to the crown of your head; each one is linked to specific parts of the body and different emotions, colors, and earth elements.

CHIROPRACTOR: A therapist who manipulates bones and joints to heal disease and/or relieve pain.

CHOLESTEROL: A fatty substance found in the body; not easily soluble, it can get converted to estrogen in our bodies.

CHROMOSOMES: The strands of DNA which carry **genes**; a set of 23 chromosomes is inherited from each parent.

COAGULATION PROFILE: A blood test that determines whether your blood coagulates normally; it can be used to rule out **von Willebrand's disease**.

COMPLETE BLOOD COUNT: See CBC.

CONSCIOUS SEDATION: A state of being tranquilized but awake during a medical procedure.

CORTISOL: A hormone that helps the body respond to stress. High cortisol levels can put wear and tear on the heart, brain, and other key organs.

CREATIVE VISUALIZATION: A technique in which visualizing what you want from life starts the process of changing your reality.

CRYOMYOLYSIS: A procedure that uses extreme cold to kill **fibroids** and their blood supply.

C-SECTION (Caesarean): Surgery to deliver a baby, involving incisions in the abdomen and uterus. In a Caesarean myomectomy, fibroids are removed after the baby is delivered via C-section.

CT-SCAN: Computed tomography. An imaging technique that uses X rays to create pictures of thin slices of the body.

CURETTE: The small spoon used to scrape the lining of the **uterus** during a D&C.

D&C (DILATION AND CURETTAGE): A procedure used to check for cancerous cells in the uterine lining; it is also sometimes used to try to control very heavy bleeding.

DANAZOL (DANOCRINE): A drug that's chemically similar to the male sex hormone testosterone; it may be prescribed to stop heavy menstrual bleeding. The side effects include an increase of male characteristics, such as growing facial hair.

DEGENERATION: When fibroids die, they're said to degenerate. This process is normal: Two-thirds of fibroids show some form of degeneration.

DES: Diethylstilbestrol. A "wonder drug" given to women to prevent miscarriage, which resulted in higher levels of cancer among the women who took it, as well as in their daughters (often known as DES daughters) and sons.

DOPPLER SCAN (TRANSVAGINAL DOPPLER VELOCIMETRY): A procedure that measures how fast the blood in your uterine arteries and related blood vessels is flowing toward your fibroids.

DYSFUNCTIONAL BLEEDING: Bleeding without an obvious physical cause.

DYSMENORRHEA: Cramps. See primary and secondary dysmenorrhea.

DYSPLASIA: Abnormal cell growths.

ECTOPIC PREGNANCY: A pregnancy that forms in the Fallopian tubes.

ENDOCRINOLOGIST: A doctor specializing in the endocrine system, including the thyroid and ovaries.

ENDOMETRIAL ABLATION: A technique used to stop abnormal uterine bleeding (AUB), one of the top reasons, after fibroids, that women get hysterectomies. Experts agree that you should not have endometrial ablation if you have fibroids.

ENDOMETRIAL BIOPSY: A test used to check for cancerous cells in the endometrium (lining of the uterus).

ENDOMETRIAL CANCER: Cancer that begins in the lining of the uterus, or endometrium.

ENDOMETRIOSIS: A condition in which pieces of the uterine lining have somehow migrated to other parts of the pelvis; symptoms include pain, difficulty during sex, irregular bleeding, and infertility. Endometriosis is second only to uterine fibroids as the most frequent cause of surgery in premenopausal women.

ENDOMETRITIS: An inflamed endometrium.

ENDOMETRIUM: The layer that surrounds the cavity of the uterus. The endometrium has two layers: a thin layer which grows new blood vessels every month, and the endometrial lining, the layer of blood that builds up every month. Also called the uterine mucosa, or the uterine lining.

ENDORPHINS: Naturally produced substances that reduce pain and improve moods.

ESTRADIOL: One of three major forms of estrogen; considered the most powerful form of natural estrogen.

ESTRIOL: One of three major forms of estrogen; estriol reaches high levels during pregnancy.

ESTROGEN: The primary female hormone, produced by the ovaries and adrenal glands, has more than twenty different variations. Estrogen plays a powerful part in keeping various parts of our bodies running smoothly, including our hearts, brains, and blood vessels. It helps us maintain healthy teeth, gums, bones, skin, and hair; increases blood flow to the vagina, creating more elasticity and lubrication. Estrogen may help reduce anxiety and depression, and maintain normal sleep cycles. Estrogen is also one of the key factors in the growth and development of **fibroids**.

ESTROGEN RECEPTORS: Special gateways into our cells which allow us to absorb estrogen.

ESTROGEN REPLACEMENT THERAPY (ERT): Synthetic estrogen, used by some women to replace natural estrogen after menopause. Women who have fibroids are generally warned against taking estrogen alone.

ESTRONE: One of three major forms of **estrogen**. Made by fat cells, estrone becomes the dominant estrogen after menopause, but can also add estrogen to your system while you're still menstruating. The heavier you are, the more estrone you produce.

FALLOPIAN TUBES (oviducts): The part of the reproductive system that provides the pathway an egg travels from the **ovaries** to the **uterus**.

FETUS: A developing baby inside the **uterus**.

FIBROIDS: Firm, well defined, round lumps of muscle, laced with blood vessels and surrounded by a tough, fibrous outer tissue. Each fibroid was once a single cell in the uterus that somehow received the wrong message about how to grow and function.

FIBROID SLOUGH: Spontaneous discharge of **fibroids** through the **vagina**.

FIBROID TUMORS: Another name for **fibroids**.

FIBROMAS: Another name for **fibroids**.

FIBROMYOMAS: Another name for **fibroids**.

FLUID SONOGRAPHY: A type of **sonogram** that involves filling your **uterus** with saline solution, to increase the size of your uterine cavity and allow better visualization of any fibroids inside the cavity.

FREE RADICALS: Molecules that trigger cell abnormalities, possibly including **fibroids**.

FSH (FOLLICLE-STIMULATING HORMONE): A hormone sent by the brain to the **ovaries** to stimulate **estrogen** production.

FUNDUS: The wide part of the **uterus**. Together, the fundus and the **isthmus** are called the "body" of the uterus, or the corpus.

G-SPOT: The coin-sized nerve center in the front wall of your vagina.

GELFOAM: An alternative to PVA, gelfoam blocks the uterine artery after UAE. Unlike PVA, gelfoam is temporary, dissolving in the body 10 to 20 days after the procedure.

GENERAL ANESTHESIA: Drugs provided before surgery, which put you in a sleep-like state so that you are aware of nothing during the operation.

GENES: Chemical units, carried by **chromosomes**, which transfer hereditary characteristics from parent to child.

GENISTEIN: A substance found in soy foods that, in tests, blocked the growth of new blood vessels.

GENETIC ABNORMALITY: A broken or damaged gene.

GNRH: Short for "gonadotropin releasing hormone," GnRH appears in your body naturally: it's a messenger hormone that tells your body to make **estrogen**.

GNRH AGONISTS: Drugs that block production of your natural **GnRH**, keeping the body from producing **estrogen**.

GYNECOLOGIST: A doctor who specializes in women's reproductive systems.

GYNECOLOGICAL ONCOLOGIST: A doctor who specializes in women's cancers.

HARMONIC SCALPEL: A surgical cutting tool that uses high frequency sound waves.

HEALTH CARE PROXY: The person who can make health care decisions on your behalf if you become incapacitated.

HEMOPHILIA: A hereditary disease in which blood does not coagulate properly.

HEPATITIS: Inflammation of the liver.

HOMEOPATHY: An alternative healing method in which illness is not considered unhealthy, but a sign of the body restoring itself to balance. Homeopathic therapy is intended to stimulate the self-healing process. Practitioners of homeopathy are called homeopaths.

HOMEOSTASIS: A state of physical and mental balance; a key goal of such alternative therapies as **Naturopathy** and **Homeopathy**.

HORMONE REPLACEMENT THERAPY (HRT): A combination of synthetic **estrogen** and **progesterone** that imitates our natural mix of hormones; prescribed to women after menopause.

HYPNOSIS: A type of visualization in which you, or your therapist, clearly state your goals and focus on them over a period of time.

HYPOMENORRHEA: Light menstrual periods at normal intervals.

HYPERMENORRHEA: Heavy menstrual periods at normal intervals.

HYPOTHALAMUS: The "central command" center in your brain, which produces hormones, and controls emotions, hunger, thirst, and other functions.

HYSTERECTOMY: Surgery that removes the **uterus**, and perhaps other parts of the reproductive system.

HYSTEROSCOPIC RESECTION: A surgical procedure done to remove small **fibroids** inside the cavity of the **uterus**. The procedure is done through the **vagina**, usually without an external incision. Also called **vaginal myomectomy**.

HYSTEROSCOPY: A procedure that can be used either for viewing the uterine lining, taking an **endometrial biopsy**, or performing a **hysteroscopic resection**.

HYSTEROSALPINGOGRAM (HSG): A test that can help determine if fibroids are blocking or constricting your **Fallopian tubes**.

IBUPROFEN: Over-the-counter medication used for pain relief. Also see **NSAID**.

IGF-1 (INSULIN-LIKE GROWTH FACTOR-1): A hormone that may have a role in fibroid growth, as well as in prostate cancer and breast cancer. IGF-1 can be produced by **BGH**, a hormone sometimes given to dairy cattle.

I-MRI-GUIDED CRYOSURGERY: A new procedure that combines improved imagery from new MRIs with **cryomyolysis**.

INDOLE-3 CARBINOL (I3C): A chemical that prevents the development of cells that respond to **estrogen**, and converts **estradiol**, a powerful form of estrogen, into the milder form called **estrone**.

INFARCTION: A condition in which the fibroid is not getting enough blood to survive and a part of it dies. This can be very painful, but not life threatening. Also see **degeneration**.

INSULIN: A hormone produced by the pancreas that helps the body process sugar.

INTRACAVITY FIBROIDS: Pedunculated fibroids that take up space inside the uterus.

INTERFERON: A drug used to treat some tumors, among other conditions. Also called interferon alpha.

INTERMENSTRUAL BLEEDING: Bleeding between menstrual periods. Also called breakthrough bleeding.

INTRAMURAL FIBROIDS: Fibroids in the uterine muscle. Also called interstitial fibroids.

ISTHMUS: The narrow passageway that connects the **cervix** and the wide part of the uterus (**fundus**).

IVF (IN-VITRO FERTILIZATION): The process of fertilizing eggs in a laboratory, most often for later implantation in the **uterus**.

KAMPO: A simplified version of TCM, developed in Japan by Buddhist monks.

KUNDALINI: The energy that unblocks and balances the **chakras**. Yoga was designed to release and stimulate kundalini.

LAMINARIA TENTS: Small tubes, made from Japanese seaweed, used to widen the **cervix** prior to a **D&C**.

LAPAROSCOPICALLY ASSISTED VAGINAL HYSTERECTOMY (LAVH): A hysterectomy that adds the element of **laparoscopy** to a vaginal procedure.

LAPAROSCOPIC MYOMECTOMY: Microsurgery used to identify and remove fibroids. It is especially effective for fibroids inside the cavity or outside the uterus.

LAPAROSCOPY: "Belly-button" surgery, during which a skilled doctor inserts various instruments through a small incision to view the pelvic organs and/or conduct surgery. Laparoscopy can be used to perform a wide variety of surgeries, including **myolysis**, **cryomyolysis**, **myomectomy**, and **hysterectomy**.

LAPAROTOMY: Open abdominal surgery; surgery takes place through an incision several inches long.

LASER ABLATION: Experimental technology which uses **MRI** imagery to guide laser fibers to **fibroids**; the fibers conduct heat up to 140 degrees Fahrenheit to coagulate fibroids. This procedure is similar to **myolysis**.

LASERS: High frequency beams of concentrated light. **Laser Surgery** is any type of surgery in which the surgeon uses lasers as a cutting tool, or in which lasers are used to destroy fibroids.

LEIOMYOMAS: Another name for **fibroids**.

LEIOMYOMATAS: Another name for **fibroids**.

LEVONORGESTREL-RELEASING IUDS: Intrauterine devices (IUDs) that release levonorgestrel (a synthetic progesterone), a contraception method that may have a side benefit of treating fibroid symptoms, notably, heavy bleeding.

LOCAL ANESTHETIC: Drugs provided prior to a surgical procedure, which allow you to remain awake but without pain during the procedure.

LPA: A test for diagnosing ovarian cancer.

LUPRON®: The strongest, and most common brand of **GnRH agonists**. Also called Lupron Depot®.

MAGNETIC RESONANCE IMAGING (MRI): Imaging technology that provides details of soft tissue and fluids deep inside the body.

MALIGNANT: Cancerous.

MEDITATION: An important component of Eastern religions, meditation can be a formal practice, or take the form of prayer, or exercise. Studies have shown that meditation techniques can help relieve the effects of chronic pain, PMS, infertility, anxiety, and depression, among other things.

MENORRHAGIA: Prolonged, heavy flow during menstrual periods.

MENOPAUSE: The time of life when hormones fall to their lowest levels.

METROMENORRHAGIA (or metrorrhagia): Heavy bleeding at unpredictable intervals.

MIFEPRISTONE (RU-486): A drug that suppresses the body's natural production of **progesterone**.

MIND-BODY TECHNIQUES: The use of conscious thought to moderate physical habits, or to learn how to explore your thoughts and feelings more deeply. Indirectly, these techniques can lead you to better physical and mental health.

MISCARRIAGE: Loss of pregnancy, usually of a fetus that is not viable outside the uterus.

MISEMBOLIZATION: The term for what happens if **PVA** particles from a **UAE** procedure get into the wrong place, where they can damage other pelvic organs.

MONOCLONAL TUMORS: Another name for **fibroids**.

MORCELLATOR: A mechanical device used during **laparoscopic surgery**, which chops your **fibroids** into small pieces and suctions them out of your body.

MONO-UNSATURATED FATS: Found in olive, canola, sesame, and peanut oils, high-oleic sunflower seed oil, high-oleic safflower seed oil.

MOXABUSTION: A TCM practice of burning herbs on or near key **acupuncture** points.

MRI: see Magnetic Resonance Imaging.

MUCOSA: A mucous membrane.

MYOFIBROMAS: Another name for **fibroids**.

MYOMAS: Another name for **fibroids**.

MYOLYSIS: A surgical technique that uses heat to kill the **fibroid** and its blood supply. Also known as **myoma coagulation**.

MYOMECTOMY: Surgery in which **fibroids** are removed and the rest of the uterus is left intact or repaired to be (almost) as good as new.

MYOMETRIUM: The uterine wall, composed of a thick layer of smooth muscle.

NAPROXEN: A non-prescription medication that can help control cramps and bleeding.

NATURAL PROGESTERONE: Made from wild yam and offered by a variety of manufacturers as a cure for fibroid symptoms, among other claims.

NATUROPATHY: An alternative healing method based on the principle that our bodies have the power to heal themselves. **Naturopaths** believe our bodies have a natural equilibrium, or **homeostasis**, which can be upset by an unhealthy lifestyle.

NECROSIS: The death of a piece of tissue.

NSAIDS: Non-steroidal anti-inflammatory drugs: primarily over-the-counter medications like aspirin, **ibuprofen,** and **naproxen.**

NUTRACEUTICALS: A term for supplements, such as vitamins and herbs, meant to add extra nutrients to a normal diet.

NATURAL HORMONE REPLACEMENT: Use of herbs and other plants that contain a weak form of **estrogen** (known as **phytoestrogens**) that you can eat, take as teas, or use as supplements.

NUTRITIONIST: A dietician or other professional specializing in nutrition.

OFF LABEL: Use of a prescription drug for conditions other than those officially approved by the FDA.

OJAS: In Ayur-Vedic medicine, the life force that keeps our bodies in balance.

OLIGOMENORRHEA: Long gaps between menstrual periods, from 41 days to 6 months.

OMEGA-6 FATTY ACIDS: Found in corn, safflower, sunflower, soybean, and sesame oils.

OOPHORECTOMY: Surgery removing one or both ovaries.

ORGANIC: A description of foods raised without chemicals.

ORGASM: See uterine orgasm.

OSTEOPOROSIS: The loss of bone mineral.

OVARIES: The organs that produce **estrogen** and **progesterone**, the ovaries house and release eggs into the **Fallopian tubes**. After **menopause**, your ovaries don't "die," but still produce tiny amounts of these hormones, continuing their beneficial effect to a small degree.

OVULATORY BLEEDING: A normal menstrual period, occurring every 21–40 days.

PAP SMEAR: A routine test to screen for cervical cancer.

PARASITIC LEIOMYOMATA: Pedunculated fibroids, growing on a stalk from the outer wall of the uterus, which outgrow their original blood supply in the **uterus** and begin to draw blood from other organs in the pelvis.

PARTIAL HYSTERECTOMY: See supracervical **hysterectomy**.

PERCUTANEOUS LASER ABLATION: A type of surgery in which special fibers, inserted through needles into a **fibroid**, are heated to over 140 degrees, killing the fibroid cells.

PEDUNCULATED FIBROIDS: Fibroids shaped like a ball on a stalk.

PERIMENOPAUSE: The stage of life beginning anywhere from five to ten years before menopause. Every woman's timing is different, but most women begin to go into perimenopause between their late thirties and late forties. This is the time when **estrogen** and **progesterone** may be most out of balance, and **fibroids** are most likely to go through growth spurts.

PHYTOESTROGENS: A form of **estrogen** that exists in plants.

THE PILL: *See* birth control pill.

PIRFENIDONE: A new drug, still in experimental testing, which may prevent the growth of **fibroid** cells.

PLACEBO: A harmless substance often used in controlled experiments to test the effect of known drugs. The belief that a placebo is real medicine may promote healing in some people; this is known as the "placebo effect."

PLACENTAL ABRUPTION: When the placenta separates from the wall of the **uterus** between the 20th and 37th weeks of pregnancy.

PLACENTA PREVIA: A condition in which the placenta tears loose, creating a raw, bleeding spot inside the **uterus**.

POLYCYSTIC OVARIES: A condition in which ovaries develop a thick outer wall, under which unreleased eggs form cysts. This condition is not known to be related to fibroids.

POLYMENORRHEA: Menstrual periods that occur at shorter than usual intervals, every 21 days or less.

POLYPS: Fleshy growths that grow from the lining of the **uterus** into the uterine cavity. Polyps are almost always **benign**.

POSTMENOPAUSE: The term used for when hormones have declined to their lowest levels, although the **ovaries** continue to produce small amounts of hormones throughout a woman's life.

POSTMENOPAUSAL BLEEDING: Bleeding occurring more than 1 year after menopause.

POSTPARTUM HEMORRHAGE: Heavy bleeding after delivery.

PRANA: See Ojas.

PREMARIN®: An estrogen replacement drug made by Wyeth-Ayerst. The contraindications for Premarin® include **fibroids**.

PREMATURE RUPTURE OF THE MEMBRANES (PROM): Tearing of the delicate and flexible membrane surrounding the unborn baby inside the uterus; in extreme cases, large **fibroids** during pregnancy can put pressure on this membrane, causing it to break open, or rupture.

PRETERM LABOR: Labor beginning before the 37th week of pregnancy.

PRIMARY DYSMENORRHEA: Cramps caused by **prostaglandins**, the hormones that make your **uterus** contract during menstruation. Most women who have primary dysmenorrhea have had it most of their lives.

PROGESTERONE: A hormone that works in partnership with **estrogen** to regulate pregnancy and our periods. It may also be a factor in **fibroid** growth.

PROLAPSE: See Uterine prolapse.

PROPHYLACTIC SURGERIES: Preventive surgery, generally in healthy people, used to avoid possible future disease.

PROSTACYCLINS: A natural substance that causes blood vessels to relax.

PROSTAGLANDINS: A substance the uterus produces, which, among other functions, promotes uterine contractions and may stimulate tumor growth.

PROTON BEAM THERAPY: Radiation treatment that can target the unhealthy cells of a tumor, while largely leaving healthy tissue alone. Right now, proton beam therapy is limited to specific centers for cancer treatment.

PVA (POLYVINYL ALCOHOL): Tiny particles, no larger than grains of salt, used to block the uterine arteries during UAE.

QI: The life force in traditional Chinese thought. Qi is made up of two equal but opposite forces called **yin** and **yang**; these need to be in balance for perfect health.

RADICAL HYSTERECTOMY: Surgery which removes the **uterus**, **cervix**, **ovaries**, and **Fallopian tubes**, as well as supporting ligaments, tissues, the upper portion of the **vagina** and, in case of cancer, the pelvic lymph nodes.

RADIOLOGIST: A doctor who specializes in the use of imaging equipment (including **sonograms** and **MRIs**) to detect and diagnose disease.

RALOXIFENE: A SERM marketed as Evista® by Eli Lilly and Co.

RECEPTORS: See Estrogen Receptors.

RECTUM: The lowest section of the large intestine, ending with the anus.

RED DEGENERATION: See Carneous (red) degeneration.

RENAL FAILURE: Failure of healthy kidneys, often a reversable condition, is called "acute renal failure." "Chronic renal failure" refers to long-term, life-threatening kidney disease.

RU-486: The so-called "abortion pill," made from **mifepristone**, an **antiprogesterone**. Tests have shown that RU-486 can reduce **fibroid** size.

SACRAL CHAKRA: The second **chakra**, and the one most related to the **uterus**. Located in the lower abdomen, the Sacral chakra energizes a range of sensual forces. Blocked or imbalanced energy in the second chakra can result in **fibroids**. Also called the Hara chakra.

SALPINGECTOMY: Surgery removing one or both **Fallopian tubes**.

SALPINGO-OOPHORECTOMY: Surgery removing one or both **Fallopian tubes** as well as one or both **ovaries**.

SALPINGITIS: Inflamed **Fallopian tubes**.

SATURATED FATS: Dietary fat, most often found in animal products such as meat, chicken with the skin, eggs, and full-fat dairy products like cheese, ice cream, and butter.

SECONDARY DYSMENORRHEA: Cramps with an obvious cause, such as **fibroids**, pelvic inflammatory disease (PID), or **endometriosis**. These cramps aren't limited to your monthly period: they also occur during intercourse, or even during times of the month when you're not menstruating.

SELECTIVE ESTROGEN RECEPTOR MODERATORS (SERMs): Also called "designer estrogens," SERMs attempt to send **estrogen** to the places in your body where it can theoretically do the most good, like your bones, heart, and blood vessels.

SEROSA: The thin, tough outer layer of the **uterus**. It protects the uterus and connects to the ligaments that support the uterus inside your pelvic cavity.

SESSILE: A fibroid in the shape of a ball.

SHBG (SEX HORMONE BINDING GLOBULIN): A substance that binds free estrogen.

SONOGRAM: A procedure used to develop a picture of the uterus, by bouncing harmless, high frequency sound waves against the pelvis. Also called **ultrasound**.

SOY: Foods made from soybeans, such as tofu and tempeh.

SPOTTING: Light, irregular menstrual flow, including light pink or brown staining.

SUBMUCOUS FIBROIDS: Fibroids that grow from the uterine lining.

SUBSEROSAL FIBROIDS: Fibroids that form on the **serosa**, or outer layer of the uterus. Also called serosal, subserous, or subperitoneal.

SUPRACERVICAL HYSTERECTOMY: Surgery that removes just the top part of your uterus (the **fundus**). You keep your **cervix**, **ovaries**, and **Fallopian tubes**. Also called **subtotal** or **partial hysterectomy**.

SURGICAL MENOPAUSE: The result of losing both ovaries during a surgical procedure; surgical menopause is both more sudden and often more severe than natural menopause, since you lose the protective effect of the hormones the ovaries produce, even in menopause.

Sutures: The stitches or staples used to close a surgical incision.

Synarel: A brand name of a **GnRH agonist**.

Tamoxifen: A SERM used to prevent breast cancer; however, it increases the risk for uterine cancer.

Tenaculum: A special forceps used to clamp open the **cervix**.

Testosterone: A primarily male hormone. Testosterone therapy for women following hysterectomy can improve sexual libido and sexual pleasure, help prevent osteoporosis, and may protect the heart and cardiovascular system.

Tocolytic: A drug used to help stop early contractions in pregnancy.

Total abdominal hysterectomy (TAH): Surgery that removes all of your reproductive organs: the **uterus**, **cervix**, both **ovaries**, and **Fallopian tubes**.

Total hysterectomy: Surgery that removes your **uterus**, including the **cervix**, but leaves your **ovaries** and **Fallopian tubes** in place. Also called simple hysterectomy, partial hysterectomy, complete hysterectomy

Traditional Chinese Medicine (TCM): Practiced for over 2,000 years, TCM is based on the concept of balancing **Qi**, the life force that flows around and through us.

Transducer: A short, wand-like instrument used as a probe during a **sonogram** to send pictures of your pelvic cavity to the computer.

Trans-fats: An especially unhealthy form of dietary fat.

Tumor: An abnormal mass of tissue growing in the body that has no useful function and grows at the expense of the body.

Ultrasound: See sonogram.

Unopposed estrogen: Estrogen that is not balanced by **progesterone**.

Ureters: The tubes that transport urine from the kidneys.

Urinary incontinence: The inability to hold back urine.

Uterine Artery Embolization (UAE): A technique used to reduce the size and symptoms of fibroids, by injecting tiny particles into the artery to reduce the blood supply to the fibroids, starving them of blood.

Uterine crowding: A condition in which fibroids share space in the uterus with a developing baby; in some women, the effect is almost like carrying twins.

Uterine Fibroid Embolization: Another name for **Uterine Artery Embolization**.

Uterine orgasm: Quick contractions of the uterine muscle, causing sexual pleasure.

Uterine prolapse: The term for when your **uterus** is forced down and into your **vagina**.

Uterine rupture: A break in the uterine wall. While this does not happen often, it is more likely to happen when large fibroids are present during pregnancy and the uterus has been weakened from incisions during a previous surgery.

Uterine scarring: Scars left by incisions from **myomectomy**, **C-section**, or other surgery affecting the uterus. Also called **Asherman's Syndrome.**

Uterine sarcoma: Cancer that starts in the muscles of the uterus.

Uterus: Sexual and reproductive organ, which plays a unique role in orgasms, provides structural support for other organs in your pelvis, and is a rich source of hormones and other natural, beneficial substances. The uterus is home for developing embryos; it is also where **fibroids** form.

VAGINA: An elastic sheath of muscle and tissue, forming a passage leading to the uterus. The vagina is anchored internally by the **cervix.**

VAGINAL HYSTERECTOMY: An operation that removes the uterus through the vagina, with no external incision.

VAGINAL MYOMECTOMY: Also called **hysteroscopic resection**, surgery that removes relatively small fibroids from inside the cavity of the uterus, via the vagina, using no external incision.

VAGINAL SONOGRAM: Shows pictures of the uterus by means of a probe inserted into the vagina.

VAGUS NERVE: A nerve which goes directly from the cervix to the brain stem, thought to be an independent pathway for the sensations of orgasm.

VASCULAR DISEASE: Disease affecting the blood vessels.

VON WILLEBRAND'S DISEASE: An inherited bleeding disorder which makes blood clot more slowly than normal: it affects up to 3 out of every hundred women (3 percent).

WAIST-TO-HIP RATIO: A measurement indicating body shape. It is found by dividing waist size by hip size: a 30-inch waist and 40-inch hips have a ratio of 0.75.

WATCH AND WAIT: The practice of observing fibroids over a period of time, postponing more aggressive treatment until symptoms or fibroid growth warrant it.

XENOESTROGENS: Man-made compounds that mimic estrogen, found in pesticides and other chemicals.

YIN AND YANG: These two forces compose **Qi**, and need to be in balance for perfect health. **Yang** is associated with heat, dryness, light, action, and expansion. **Yin** is cold, damp, dark, and quiet; it's associated with the earth, interior, and deficiency.

YOGA: Originally developed as a component of **Ayur-Veda**, yoga is a system of mind-body training, relying on specific exercises, breathwork, and meditation to release and stimulate **kundalini,** the energy that unblocks and balances the chakras.

ZOFRAN: A drug used by anesthesiologists to prevent post-operative nausea.

ZOLADEX: A brand name **GnRH agonist.**

Selected Resources

Find out more about fibroids

Agency for Health Care Research & Quality: *www.ahcpr.gov*.

America OnLine: women's health, Tumors, Fibroids, and Cysts bulletin board: *www.aol.com*.

Center for Uterine Fibroids at Brigham and Women's Hospital in Boston: *www.fibroids.net*, one of the top research centers for fibroids.

CenterWatch Patient Notification Subscriber: a free service to notify patients, professionals, and patient advocates of news about clinical trials and drugs in research. Subscribe at *www.centerwatch.com/patient/pns/patemail.asp*.

Clinical Trials, National Library of Medicine: *www.clinicaltrials.gov*.

Clinical Trials, National Institutes of Health: *www.nih.gov/health*.

The Fibroid Place: *www.delphi.com/fibroids/start*.

Fibroid Network/Sisternetwork: 27 Old Gloucester Street, London, WC1N 3XX, UK. e-mail: welcome@fibroidnetwork.com, website: *www.fibroidnetwork.com*, *www.sisternetwork.com*.

Fibroids/UK, Ireland, online discussion group:
www.smartgroups.com/groups/fibroids.
The Fibroid Zone: *www.fibroidzone.com.*
Management of Uterine Fibroids: report by the Agency for Healthcare
Research and Quality. A lengthy summary is available online at
www.ahrq.gov/clinic/utersumm.htm. The full report is available online at
www.ahrq.gov/clinic/epcix.htm, or by calling 1-800-358-9295. Ask for "Evidence Report/Technology Assessment No. 34, Management of Uterine
Fibroids (AHRQ Publication No. 01-E052)."
Medscape Women's Health: *www.medscape.com*; search for recent articles,
studies.
National Institutes of Health, Office of Research on Women's Health:
www4.od.nih.gov/orwh.
The National Library of Medicine's Medline® and Pre-Medline® Databases:
www.medportal.com; search for recent articles, studies.
ObGyn Net: *www.obgyn.com.* Probably the most comprehensive source of
women's health information on the web, with opportunities to network
with other women as well as doctors.
Waypages: *www.waypages.com/health*, links to several health search engines.

Dealing with symptoms

Lark, Susan M., M.D. *Dr. Susan Lark's Heavy Menstrual Flow & Anemia Self
Help Book.* San Francisco: Celestial Arts, 1995.
Inlet Medical, online discussion groups: *www.inletmedical.org/forum/
default.asp.*

Healthy nutrition

Lark, Susan M., M.D. *Fibroid Tumors & Endometriosis Self Help Book.* San
Francisco: Celestial Arts, 1995.
Food and Fitness Advisor: 1-800-829-2505 for subscription information.
Natural Health: www.naturalhealth1.com, or 1-800-526-8440 for subscription
information.
Tufts University: *www.navigator.tufts.edu*: search engine for numerous nutri-
tional resources.

Mind-body medicine, stress reduction

Domar, Alice D., Ph.D. and Henry Dreher. *Healing Mind, Healthy Woman:
Using the Mind-Body Connection to Manage Stress and Take Control of
Your Life.* New York: A Delta Book/Dell Publishing, 1996.
Ellwood, Robert. *Finding the Quiet Mind.* Wheaton, IL: The Theosophical
Publishing House, 1987.

Gawain, Shakti. *Creative Visualization*. New York: A Bantam New Age Book, 1978, 1982.

Gawain, Shakti. *Creative Visualization*. New York: A Bantam New Age Book, 1978, 1982.

Mind/Body Health Newsletter; The Center for Health Services, c/o ISHK Book Service, P.O. Box 381069, Cambridge, MA 02238-1069, 1-800-222-4745 for subscription information.

Estrogen, xenoestrogens, and HRT

Love, Susan M., M.D. with Karen Lindsay. *Dr. Susan Love's Hormone Book: Making Informed Choices About Menopause*. New York: Times Books, 1997.

Steinman, David and Samuel S. Epstein, M.D. *The Safe Shopper's Bible*. New York: Macmillan, 1995. For information on the safety of household cleaners.

Environmental Defense Fund: *www.scorecard.org*. Check out names of chemicals you may be working with to see if they're considered endocrine or reproductive threats.

Environmental Protection Agency: 703-305-5017; *www.epa.gov*, for information about pesticide programs.

Lupron, TAP Pharmaceuticals: *www.lupron.com*.

Mothers & Others for a Livable Planet: 888-ECO-INFO, *www.mothers.org*, for information on safe plastic products.

Kellar, Casey. *Natural Cleaning for Your Home: 95 Pure and Simple Recipes*. Lark Books, 1998. For natural cleaning and stain fighting.

The National Lupron Victims Network: *www.lupronvictims.com*

Health records

WebMD: My Health Record, *my.webmd.com/my_health_record*.

Insurance issues: checking on coverage

Orin, Rhonda D. *Making Them Pay: How to Get the Most from Health Insurance and Managed Care*. New York: St. Martin's, Griffin.

www.ehealthinsurance.com compares the rates of fifty-six carriers representing more than 4,000 plans.

Health Insurance Portability and Accountability Act of 1996: *www.hcfa.gov/medicaid/HIPAA/content/q&a-con.asp*.

McCullough, Campbell & Lane, Attorneys at Law, *www.mcandl.com*, online publication *Summary Of United States Medical Malpractice Law*.

Medical Insurance Bureau: *www.MIB.com*, collects information from your medical insurance company each time you file a claim; order a copy of your report for a small fee.

Center for Patient Advocacy
  1350 Beverly Road, Suite 108
  McLean, VA 22101
  703-748-0400 or 800-846-7444
  Fax: 703-748-0402
  www.patientadvocacy.org.
Consumer Coalition for Quality Health Care
  1101 Vermont Avenue NW, Suite 1001
  Washington, DC 20005
  202-789-3606
  www.consumers.org.
Patient Advocate Foundation
  753 Thimble Sholas Boulevard #B
  Newport News, VA 23606
  757-873-6668
  www.patientadvocate.org

Alternative medicine

Nissim, Rina. *Natural Healing in Gynaecology: A manual for women.* London: Pandora, 1996.
Weil, Andrew, Dr. *Dr. Andrew Weil's Self-Healing Newsletter*, 42 Pleasant St., Watertown, MA 02472. Phone: 800-523-3296.
Woodham, Anne and Dr. David Peters. *Encyclopedia of Healing Therapies.* New York: Dorling Kindersley, 1997.
Alternative Health News Online: *www.altmedicine.com.*
The Alternative Medicine Home Page: *www.alternativemedicine.com.* Numerous links for acupuncture, homeopathy, naturopathy, and other alternative care information resources.
America OnLine/Alt.Med: *www.aol.com*, search health/alternative medicine channel for fibroids.
Medformation: *www.medformation.com*, a collection of alternative medicine links.
NCCAM, the National Center for Complementary and Alternative Medicine: part of the NIH, *nccam.nih.gov.*

Herbs

Graedon, Joe and Teresa Graedon. *The People's Pharmacy Guide to Home and Herbal Remedies.* NY: St. Martin's Griffin, 2001.
Hadady, Letha. *Asian Health Secrets.* NY: Three Rivers Press, 1996.
Harrar, Sari and Sara Altshul O'Donnell. *The Woman's Book of Healing Herbs.* Emmaus,PA: Rodale Press, Inc., 1999.

McIntyre, Anne. *The Complete Woman's Herbal: A Manual of Healing Herbs and Nutrition for Personal Well-Being and Family Care.* New York: Henry Holt & Co., 1995.

Tyler, Varro, M.D. and James E. Robbers. *Tyler's Herbs of Choice.* Haworth Press, 1999.

Tyler, Varro, M.D. and Steven Foster. *Tyler's Honest Herbal.* Haworth Press, 1999.

Medwatch, a monitoring program of the Food and Drug Administration for all suspected adverse reactions to herbal products. Call the toll-free number, 800-FDA-1088, or contact the program on line at *www.fda.gov/medwatch.*

The National Institutes of Health lists information on dietary supplements, including herbal products, at *www.nal.usda.gov/fnic/IBIDS.*

TCM

www.acupuncture.com: a resource for multiple links.

Qi: The Journal of Traditional Eastern Health and Fitness: *www.qi-journal.com*

American Association of Acupuncture and Oriental Medicine
433 Front Street
Catasauqua, PA 18032
610-266-1433 or 888-500-7999
www.aaom.org, for information on TCM and Kampo

American College of Traditional Chinese Medicine
455 Arkansas Street
San Francisco, CA 94107
415-282-7600
fax: 415-282-0856
www.actcm.edu.

Foundation for Traditional Chinese Medicine (UK)
122A Acomb Road
York YO2 4EY, England
www.demon.co.uk/acupuncture/ftcm.html.

National Commission for the Certification of Acupuncturists
1424 16th Street, NW
Suite 601
Washington, DC 20036
202-232-1404
www.nccaom.org.

Hypnosis

Infinity Institute International, Inc.: *www.infinityinst.com*/faq.html, offers FAQs and links.

Homeopathy

Cummings, Stephen, M.D. and Dana Ullman. *Everybody's Guide to Homeo-pathic Medicine*. New York: Tarcher/Putnam, 1991.
Ullman, Dana, MPH. *The Consumer's Guide to Homeopathy*. New York: Tarcher/Putnam, 1996.
Homeopathy Internet Resources: *www.holisticmed.com/www/ homeopathy.html, numerous links.*
National Center for Homeopathy
    801 North Fairfax
    Suite 306
    Alexandria, VA 22314
    877-624-0613 or 703-548-7790
    fax: 703-548-7792
    www.homeopathic.org
    Provides directories of homeopathic pharmacies and practitioners.

Naturopathy

National College of Naturopathic Medicine: the oldest accredited school of natural medicine in North America: *www.ncnm.edu.*
American Association of Naturopathic Physicians
    8201 Greensboro Drive
    Suite 300
    McLean, VA 22102
    703-610-9037
    www.naturopathic.org.

Chakras

Angelo, Jack. *Hands-On Healing*. VT: Healing Arts Press, 1997.
Gilekson, Jim. *Energy Healing: A Pathway to Inner Growth*. New York: Marlowe & Co., 2000.
Villoldo, Alberto, Ph.D. *Shaman, Healer, Sage*. New York: Harmony Books, 2000.

Ayur-Veda

Lonsdorf, Nancy, M.D., Veronica Butler, M.D., and Melanie Brown, Ph.D. *A Woman's Best Medicine: Health, Happiness and Long Life Through Maharishi Ayur-Veda*. New York: Jeremy P. Tarcher/Putnam, 1995.

The Ayurvedic Institute
11311 Menaul NE
Albuquerque, NM 87112
505-291-9698
fax: 505-294-7572
www.ayurveda.com.

Pregnancy

Curtis, Glade B., M.D. *Your Pregnancy: Questions and Answers.* FACOG,
Fisher Books, 1995.
Eisenberg, Arlene, Heidi E. Murkoff, and Sandee E. Hathaway, B.S.N. *What
to Expect When You're Expecting.* New York: Workman Publishing, 1991.
Hales, Dianne, and Timothy R.B. Johnson, M.D. *Intensive Caring: New Hope
for High-Risk Pregnancy.* New York: Crown Publishers, Inc., 1990.
Hutcherson, Hilda, M.D. with Margaret Williams. *Having Your Baby: A
Guide for African-American Women.* New York: One World/Ballantine
Books, 1997.
Atlanta Reproductive Health Center: *www.ivf.com.* Look for Mark Perloe,
M.D., and Linda Gail's article, "Miracle Babies and Other Happy Endings."

Miscarriage

Friedman, Lynn, M.D. with Irene Daria. *A Woman Doctor's Guide to
Miscarriage.* New York: Hyperion, 1996.
National SHARE Office
St. Joseph Health Center
300 First Capitol Drive
St Charles, MO 63301
800-821-6819 or 314-947-6164
fax: 636-947-7486
www.nationalshareoffice.com.
Pregnancy and infant loss support.
Pregnancy and Infant Loss Center
1421 East Wayzata Boulevard
Wayzata, MN 55391
612-473-9372
fax: 952-473-8978
www.pilc.org.

Infertility

RESOLVE, the nationwide network for infertile couples. National helpline:
617-623-0744, *www.resolve.org.*

How do you know if your doctor is a specialist?

American Board of Medical Specialities, lists whether a doctor is board certified: *www.abms.org.*

American Board of Obstetrics and Gynecology: *www.abog.org.*

American College of Obstetricians and Gynecologists: *www.acog.org.*

FDA Directory of State and Local Officials, 2001, *www.fda.gov/ora/fed_state/directorytable.htm,* immensely comprehensive information on state health offices and officials to contact.

The Federation of State Medical Boards: www.fsmb.org, contact information for state medical boards.

Health Grades: *www.healthgrades.com,* for information about doctors and hospitals.

Pub Med: Read your doctor's articles, if any, at *www.ncbi.nlm.nih.gov/entrez/query.fcgi.*

Information about cancer

The Association of Cancer Online Resources, Inc.: *www.acor.org,* a gateway to online cancer support groups used by more than 67,000 members.

CancerNet, a service of the National Cancer Institute/NIH, includes a variety of sources to help meet your cancer information needs: 800-4-CANCER, *cancernet.nci.nih.gov.*

The Gynecological Cancers Online Support Discussion Group; get on their discussion list by contacting *owner-gyn-onc@listserv.acor.org.*

OncoLink, *www.oncolink.org.* Look for NCI/PDQ Patient Statement: Uterine Sarcoma.

Helpful information before surgery

Hartman, Lauren. *Solutions: The Woman's Crisis Handbook.* New York: Houghton Mifflin, 1997. Practical advice, including how to handle problems at work due to medical crises.

Family Medical Leave Act, from the U.S. Department of Labor, *www.dol.gov/dol/esa/fmla.htm.*

Uterine Artery Embolization (UAE)

Embolization support group. E-mail discussion group. To subscribe, send an empty message to embo-subscribe@yahoogroups.com.

The Fibroid Corner, from Delaware Valley Imaging, one of the first UAE practices in the U.S. (1996), *www.fibroidcorner.com.*

The Fibroid Embolization Center at the NY United Hospital Medical Center
    406 Boston Post Road
    Port Chester, NY 10573
    877-934-3628 (toll free) or 914-934-3355
    www.uhmc.com/fibroid.htm.
Georgetown Medical School
Vascular & Interventional Radiology
    Department of Radiology
    Ground Floor, CCC Building
    Georgetown University Medical Center
    Washington, DC
    202-784-3420
    www.dml.georgetown.edu/depts/radiology.
Society of Cardiovascular & Interventional Radiology (SCVIR)
    10201 Lee Highway
    Suite 500,
    Fairfax, VA 22030
    800-488-7284 or 703-691-1805
    fax: 703-691-1855
    e-mail: info@scvir.org
    www.scvir.org.
    Information on UAE; national doctor finder.

Myomectomy

Stringer, Nelson H., M.D. *Uterine Fibroids: What Every Woman Needs to
    Know.* IL; Physicians & Scientists Publishing Co., Inc., 1996.
    www.fibroids.com for info on laparoscopic myomectomy.
INCIID
    InterNational Council on Infertility Information Dissemination
    P.O. Box 6836
    Arlington, VA 22206
    703-379-9178
    fax: 703-379-1593
    e-mail: INCIIDinfo@inciid.org.
    www.inciid.org.
Comprehensive information on infertility and reproductive surgery.
West, Stanley, M.D. *The Hysterectomy Hoax.* New York: Doubleday, 1994.
Intradesign, *www.intradesign.com/forums*, bulletin boards for discussions with
    other women about myomectomy and related topics.
TTCMyomectomy (trying to conceive after myomectomy), online discussion
    group: *www.egroups.com/group/ttcmyomectomy.*

Hysterectomy

Cutler, Winnifred B. *Hysterectomy, Before and After*. New York: Harper & Row, 1988.

The HERS Foundation (Hysterectomy Educational Resources and Services)
422 Bryn Mawr Avenue
Bala Cynwyd, PA 19004
610-667-7757
fax: 610-667-8096
www.hersfoundation.com.
Information about fibroid treatments; physician referrals.

Hysterectomy support group. Send a message to *hysterectomysupport@egroups.com* to join e-mail discussion group.

The Hysterectomy Association, UK: *www.hysterectomy-association.org.uk*.

Sans Uteri: *www.findings.net/sans-uteri.html*, a comprehensive site discussing first-hand reactions to hysterectomy, both pro and con, from women who've had one. Read discussions online; subscribe to their e-mail discussion group for $12 per year.

Staying healthy, staying informed

Angier, Natalie. *Woman: An Intimate Geography*. New York: Houghton Mifflin, 1999.

Northrup, Christiane, M.D. *Women's Bodies, Women's Wisdom*. New York: Bantam Books, 1994.

Black Women's Health: online discussion group at *www.delphi.com/bwhhealth/start*.

Canadian Women's Health Network: *www.cwhn.ca*.

National Library of Medicine: *www.nlm.nih.gov*.

National Women's Health Information Center (NWHIC). 800-994-WOMAN, *www.4woman.org*. Provides access to thousands of Federal and non-Federal organizations and publications.

New York Times: www.nytimes.com/women.

The Office of Minority Health Resource Center, U.S. Department of Health and Human Services. Phone: 800-444-6472, *www.omhrc.gov*.

Hoffman, Eileen, M.D. *Our Health, Our Lives: A Revolutionary Approach to Total Health Care for Women*. New York: Pocket Books, 1995.

National Black Women's Health Project
1211 Connecticut Avenue, NW
Suite 310
Washington, DC 20036
202-835-0117
www.nationalblackwomenshealthproject.org.

National Institutes of Health
Office of Research on Women's Health
Building 1, Room 201
9000 Rockville Pike
Bethesda, MD 20892-0161
301-402-1770
fax: 301-402-1798
www4.od.nih.gov/orwh.
Office of Research on Minority Health
6707 Democracy Boulevard
Suite 800, MSC 5465
Bethesda, MD 20892-5465
301-402-1366
fax: 301-480-4049
www1.od.nih.gov/ormh/main.html.
Public Citizen, The Health Research group: *www.citizen.org.*
Reuters Health: *www.reutershealth.com/frame2/eline.html.*
Sexual Health Network: *www.sexualhealth.com.*
Society for Women's Health Research
1828 L Street, NW
Suite 625
Washington, DC 20036
202-223-8224
fax: 202-833-3472
www.womens-health.org.
Thrive OnLine: *thriveonline.oxygen.com.* See my article at
*http://thriveonline.oxygen.com/medical/herhealth/herhero/fibroids.
johanna.html.*
USA Today, Health News: *www.usatoday.com/news/healthscience/hsfront.htm.*
WebMD: *www.webmd.com*, or *http://mywebmd.com.* Click on the women's
health link for boards and information.
Women's Health Advocate Newsletter. WHA, P.O.B. 420235, Palm Coast, FL.
32142-0235, 800-829-5876 for subscription information.

Help in finding reputable websites

The American Accreditation Health Care Commission: *www.urac.org*, has
issued criteria that health sites must meet to win its "seal of approval."
Kaiser Permanente created a site listing favorites of more than 4,000 consumers, along with evaluation by healthcare professionals: Health
Information Check-Up site: *www.kp.org/hicheckup/consumer/
consumer_frameset.html.*
California HealthCare Foundation:
http://ehealth.chcf.org/view.cfm?section=Industry&itemID=3973 to see
results of Rand Corporation study on standards used for evaluating clinical information on any health site.

And if you still want more . . .

Google: *www.google.com*, my (and lots of other people's) favorite search engine.

Start your own discussion group using the Yahoo/eGroup service. Instructions can be found at http://groups.yahoo.com.

Notes

Day 1

*Agency for Healthcare Research and Quality. *Management of Uterine Fibroids.* Summary, Evidence Report/Technology Assessment: Number 34. AHRQ Publication No. 01-E051 (January 2001).

Barnes and Noble Concise Medical Dictionary. New York: Barnes and Noble Books, 1995.

*Brody, J.E. *The New York Times Book of Health.* New York: Times Books, 1997.

*Center for Uterine Fibroids, *www.fibroids.net*.

*"Disorders of the Uterus: Leiomyomata Uteri." *Journal of Obstetrics & Gynecology* 8/98.

*"Fibroids: Assessing the options." *Women's Health Advocate* 3(5) (July 1996): 4–6.

*The Fibroid Embolization Center at the NY United Hospital Medical Center, *www.uhmc.com/fibroid.htm*.

*Harrison-Woolrych, M. et al. "Fibroid growth in response to high-dose progestogen." *Fertility & Sterility* 64(1) (July 1995): 191–192.

*Kjerulff, K.H. et al. "Uterine leiomyomas: Racial differences in severity, symptoms, and age at diagnosis." *Journal of Reproductive Medicine* (July 1996): 483–490.

*Li, S. et al. "Decreased expression of Wnt7a mRNA is inversely associated with the expression of estrogen receptor-alpha in human uterine leiomyoma." *Journal of Clinical Endocrinology & Metabolism* b8 6(1) (January 2001): 454–457.

*Lumsden, M.A. et al. "The binding of steroids to myometrium and leiomyomata (fibroids) in women treated with the gonadotrophin-releasing hormone agonist Zoladex" (ICI 118630), *Journal of Endocrinology* 121(2) (May 1989): 389–396.

*Marshall, L.M. et al. "Variation in the incidence of uterine leiomyoma among premenopausal women by age and race." *Obstetrics and Gynecology* 90(6) (December 1997): 967–973.

*Ochiai, K. et al. "Morbidity of uterine fibroids in Japanese women." *Obstetrics and Gynecology* 95(4 Suppl 1) (April 2000): 532.

*Olden, K. Director, National Institute of Environmental Health Sciences, National Institutes of Health, Department of Health and Human Services, FY 1996 Budget request for NIH/NIEHS, Testimony, *www.hhs.gov/progorg/asl/testify/t950314b.txt.* 3/14/95.

Oxford American Dictionary. New York: Heald Colleges Edition, Avon Books, 1980:993.

*Parker, W.H. *A Gynecologist's Second Opinion*. New York: Plume Books, 1996.

*Sato, F. et al. "Body fat distribution and uterine leiomyomas." *Epidemiology* (August 1998):176–180.

*Shikora, S.A. et al. "Relationship between obesity and uterine leiomyomata." *Nutrition* 7(4) (July–August 1991): 251–255.

*Siccardi, D.C. "Leiomyomas," Obstetrics & Gynecology, Medstudents, *www.medstudents.com.br/ginob/ginob6.htm.*

*Snieder, H. et al. "Genes control the cessation of a woman's reproductive life: a twin study of hysterectomy and age at menopause." *Journal of Clinical Endocrinological Metabolism* 83(6) (June 1998): 1875–1880.

*Spirtas, R., Chief, Contraceptive and Reproductive Evaluation Branch, National Institute of Child Health and Human Development, Testimony before the Presidential Advisory Committee on Gulf War Veterans' Illnesses, Epidemiology of and Research on Infertility, Subfertility, Fetal Loss, and Birth Defects in the United States, Public And Panel Meeting on Reproductive Health of Gulf War Veterans, Monday, June 17, 1996, Seattle, Washington.

*Stewart, E.A. et al. "Leiomyoma-related bleeding: a classic hypothesis updated for the molecular era." *Human Reproduction Update* vol. 2, no. 4 (1996): 295–306.

*"Uterine Fibroids," National Institutes of Health, *www.nih.gov/nichd/html/news/uterine.htm.*

*"Uterine Leiomyomata." *ACOG Educational Bulletin* Number 192 (May 1994).

Day 2

*Chopelas, A. "Fibroid Study and Research Program: Causes, Symptoms, Relief and Possible Solutions," 1997, originally published on Intradesign.com.

*Center for Uterine Fibroids, *www.fibroids.net.*

*Clayman, C. ed. *The Human Body*. New York: Dorling Kindersley Ltd., 1995.

*Consumer Patient Radiation Health and Safety Acts: SDMS Position Statement, Women's Health Forum, *www.ob-gyn.net.*

*Ferrini, R. "Screening Asymptomatic Women for Ovarian Cancer, American College of Preventive Medicine Practice Policy." *American Journal of Preventive Medicine* 13(6) (November/December 1997): 444–446.

*The Fibroid Embolization Center, *www.uhmc.com/fibroid.htm.*

*Goldfarb, H.A. et al. *The No-Hysterectomy Option: Your Body—Your Choice*. New York: John Wiley & Sons, 1997.

*"Naturally-Occurring Antibiotic Found In Female Urinary/Reproductive Tract." *The Doctor's Guide*, *www.pslgroup.com/dg/6C872.htm.* 4/15/98.

*Nuland, S.B. *The Mysteries Within*. New York: Simon & Schuster, 2000.

*Parker, W.H. *A Gynecologist's Second Opinion*. New York: Plume Books, 1996.

*Parsons, A.K. "Saline Infusion Sonohysterography." *Medica Mundi* 45/2, July 2001.

*Pollard, R.R. et al. "Prolapsed cervical myoma after uterine artery embolization. A case report." *Journal of Reproductive Medicine* 46(5) (May 2001): 499–500.

*Siccardi, D.C. "Leiomyomas," Obstetrics & Gynecology, Medstudents, *www.medstudents.com/br/ginob/ginob6.htm.*

*Stewart, E.A. et al. "Leiomyoma-related bleeding: a classic hypothesis updated for the molecular era." *Human Reproduction Update* vol. 2, no. 4 (1996): 295–306.

*"Uterine Fibroids," National Institutes of Health, *www.nih.gov/nichd/html/news/uterine.htm.*

*"Uterine Leiomyomata," *ACOG Educational Bulletin* Number 192 (May 1994).

*"Uterine Myomas (Fibroids)," Medfem Clinic website, *www.medfem.co.za/fibroids.ht.*

Day 3

*Baker, K. "Anemia, What every woman should know." AltMed, Health Channel, *www.aol.com.*

*Broder, M.S. et al. "Uterine Artery Embolization: A Systematic Review of the Literature and Proposal for Research." Santa Monica, CA: The Rand Corp.: 20.

*Center for Uterine Fibroids, *www.fibroids.net.*

*Chopelas, A. "Fibroid Study and Research Program: Causes, Symptoms, Relief and Possible Solutions." 1997, originally published on Intradesign.com.

*Courban, D. et al. "Acute renal failure in the first trimester resulting from uterine leiomyomas." *American Journal of Obstetrics and Gynecology* (August 1997): 472.

*"Dysfunctional Uterine Bleeding." GenneX Healthcare Technologies, *www.womenshealth.org/ask/hyst.ht.*

*"Fertility, Family Planning, and Women's Health: New Data from the 1995 National Survey of Family Growth." Vital and Health Statistics, Centers for Disease Control and Prevention, National Center for Health Statistics, U.S. Department of Health Human Services, Series 23 No. 19 (May 1997): 7.

*The Fibroid Embolization Center, *www.uhmc.com/fibroid.htm.*

*Goodman, A. "Abnormal Genital Tract Bleeding." *Clinical Cornerstone* 3(1) (2000): 25–35.

*Hale, E. "Taming Menstrual Cramps." *FDA Consumer Magazine,* *www.fda.gov/bbs/topics/CONSUMER/CON00004.html. 6/91.*

*Hales, D. et al. *Intensive Caring: New Hope for High-Risk Pregnancy.* New York: Crown Publishers, Inc., 1990.

*Hasan, F. et al. "Uterine leiomyomata in pregnancy." *International Journal of Gynaecology & Obstetrics* 34(1) (January 1991): 45–48.

*Hurd, S., Acting Director, National Institute of Nursing Research, National Institutes of Health, Department of Health and Human Services, House Appropriations Labor, Health and Human Services and Education FY96 Labor-HHS Appropriations, March 22, 1995, *www.hhs.gov/progorg/asl/testify/t950322c.txt.*

*Hutcherson, H. et al. *Having Your Baby: A Guide for African-American Women.* New York: One World/Ballantine Books, 1997.

*Ince, S. "What your period reveals about your health," *Redbook* 194(1A) (January 2000): 34, 38, 40.

*Lauersen, N. et al. *Listen To Your Body.* New York: Berkley Books, 1982.

*Levie, M., Uterine Artery Embolization: Laparoscopic Myomectomy, XVI World Congress of the International Federation of Gynecology and Obstetrics, Women's Health Conference Summaries, Medscape 2000.

*Maderas, L. et al. *Womancare.* New York: Avon Books, 1981.

*Siccardi, D.C. "Leiomyomas," Obstetrics & Gynecology, Medstudents, *www.medstudents.com.br/ginob/ginob6.htm.*

*Stewart, E.A. et al. "Leiomyoma-related bleeding: a classic hypothesis updated for the molecular era." *Human Reproduction Update* vol. 2, no. 4 (1996): 295–306.

*Stewart, F. et al. *Understanding Your Body.* New York: Bantam Books, 1987.

*Society for Women's Health Research. "Survey Shows Two-Thirds of Women are Unaware of Alternatives to Hysterectomy for Treating Excessive Menstrual Bleeding." *www.womens-health.org, 11/28/00.*

*"Uterine Leiomyomata." *ACOG Educational Bulletin* Number 192 (May 1994).

*"Uterine Fibroids," National Institutes of Health, *www.nih.gov/nichd/html/news/uterine.htm.*

*West, S. *The Hysterectomy Hoax.* New York: Doubleday, 1994.

Day 4

*Bunge, D. "Heavy periods may signal a little-known problem." *Woman's Day* (May 15, 2001): 57.

*Center for Uterine Fibroids, *www.fibroids.net*.

*Goodman, A. "Abnormal Genital Tract Bleeding." *Clinical Cornerstone*, 3(1) (2000): 25–35.

*Kadir, R.A. et al. "Frequency of inherited bleeding disorders in women." *The Lancet* 351 (1998): 485–489.

*Kotulak, R. *Inside the Brain*. Kansas City: Andrews and McMeel, 1996.

*Lipman, J.C. "Uterine Artery Embolization for the Treatment of Symptomatic Uterine Fibroids: A Review." *Applied Radiology* 29(7) (2000): 15–20.

*Perlmutter, C. "Just Say Wait A Minute." *Prevention* (January 1, 1998).

*"Sharing Feelings Can Help Breast Cancer Survivors." *Journal of Behavioural Medicine* 24 (2001): 231–245.

*"Treatment of Common Non-Cancerous Uterine Conditions: Issues for Research." AHCPR Pub. No. 95–0067 (July 1995).

*Weinstein, K. *Living With Endometriosis*. Reading, MA: Addison-Wesley Publishing Company, 1987.

Day 5

*Baird, D.D. Epidemiology Branch, Environmental Diseases and Medicine Program, Division of Intramural Research, National Institute of Environmental Health Sciences, Epidemiology web page.

*Baker, K. "Anemia, What every woman should know," AltMed, Health Channel, AOL.

*Boyd et al. "Women's Health Research at NIEHS." *Environmental Health Perspectives* no.2/vol. 101(June 1993).

*Brody, J.E. *The New York Times Book of Health*. New York: Times Books, 1997.

*Chopelas, A. "Fibroid Study and Research Program: Causes, Symptoms, Relief and Possible Solutions." 1997, originally published on Intradesign.com.

*"Essential Fatty Acids: Getting Back in Balance." *Women's Health Advocate* (May 1998): 4–6.

*Goldstein, S.R. et al. *The Estrogen Alternative*. New York: G.P. Putnam's Sons, 1998.

*LaMont, S. "Fiber, Fat and Breast Cancer Prevention." AltMed, Health Channel, AOL.

*Lark, S.M. et al. *Fibroid Tumors & Endometriosis*. Berkeley, CA: Celestial Arts, 1993.

*Love, S.M. et al. *Dr. Susan Love's Hormone Book*. New York: Times Books, 1997.

*McDougall, J.A. Hormone Dependent Diseases, *www.drmc-dougall.com.*
*McKenzie, J. "Is Cow's Milk Additive Safe?" Consumer Group Launches Action Against FDA, *abcnews.com.* 12/15/98.
*"Monitoring for Residues in Food Animals." FDA Center for Veterinary Medicine Communications and Education Branch, D.H.H.S. Pub. no. (FDA), 94–6001.
*Northrup, C. *Women's Bodies, Women's Wisdom.* New York: Bantam Books 1994.
*Pettus, E. "Can breast cancer be prevented?" *Country Living's Healthy Living,* (January 1999): 62.
*Regush, N. "You Say Tomato, I Say IGF-1." Second Opinion, *abcnews.com.* 12/17/00.
*Ross, R.K. et al. "Risk factors for uterine fibroids: reduced risk associated with oral contraceptives." *BMJ* (Clin Res Ed) 293(6543) (August 9, 1986): 359–362.
*"Soy Intake May Reduce Risk of Uterine Cancer—New Cancer Research Study." *www.pslgroup.com/dg/36266.htm.* 8/29/97.
*Stoddard, M.N. "Official Statement of Aspertame Consumer Safety Network to: President's Council on Food Safety Hearing," *http:web2/airmail/.net/marystod/council.htm,* 12/8/98.
*Weil, A. "The Sugar Buster's Diet." *Dr. Andrew Weil's Self-Healing,* 10/98:7.

Day 6

*"Acetaminophen may lower estrogen level." *Fertility and Sterility.* 70 (August 4, 1998): 371–373.
*"Dysmenorrhea (Menstrual Pain)." Alternative Medicine, *thriveonline.oxygen.com.*
*Golan, R. *Optimal Wellness.* New York: Ballantine Books, 1995.
*Keville, K. et al. "Reproductive System." Aromatherapy, HealthWorld Online, *www.healthy.net.*
*Lark, S.M. *Fibroid Tumors & Endometriosis.* Berkeley, CA: Celestial Arts, 1993.
*Lawless, J. *The Encyclopedia of Essential Oils.* New York: Barnes and Noble Books.
*Martin, R.W. "Tumors, Cysts, Fibroids, Cancer: Is Your Wood Overgrown?" AltMed, Health Channel, *www.aol.com.*
*"Uterine Fibroids," NIH pub 0051, *www.nih.gov/nichd/html/publications.html.*
*"Vitamin E: Extra protection for your health." *Food & Fitness Advisor.* (February 2000): 3.
*Weil, A. *Natural Health, Natural Medicine.* Boston, MA: Houghton Mifflin Company, 1995.
*Woodham, A. et al. *Encyclopedia of Healing Therapies.* London: Dorling Kindersley, 1997.

Day 7

*McDougall, J.A. Hormone Dependent Diseases, *www.drmc-dougall.com.*
*Ross, R.K. et al. "Risk factors for uterine fibroids: reduced risk associated with oral contraceptives." *British Medical Journal* (Clin Res Ed) 293(6543) (August 9, 1986): 359–362.

Week 2

*Begley, S. "Understanding Perimenopause." *Newsweek* Special Issue (spring/summer 1999), *www.newsweek.com/ nw-srv/printed/special/wh99/ch2/wh09_2.htm*
*Boyd et al. "Women's Health Research at NIEHS." *Environmental Health Perspectives* vol. 1, no. 2, (June 1993).
*"CDC and NIH Join in Testing Exposure of Americans to Environmental Estrogens and Other Chemicals." NIEHS PR #27-97, 11/24/97. www.niehs.nih.gov/oc/news/cdrev.htm
*Collins F., Director, National Center for Human Gene Research, Klausner R., Director, National Cancer Institute, Olden K., Director, National Institute of Environmental Health Sciences Testimony: "Cancer, Genetics, and the Environment," Department Of Health And Human Services, National Institutes of Health, before the Senate Committee on Labor and Human Resources. (March 6, 1996).
*Cooper, A. et al. "Systemic absorption of progesterone from Progest cream in postmenopausal women," *The Lancet* 351 (1998): 1255–1256.
*Drury, K. "Fighting Fibroids," *Vegetarian Times* (September 2000) :92
*Eldar-Geva, T. et al. "Other medical management of uterine fibroids." *Baillieres Clinical Obstetrics and Gynecology* 2(2) (June 1998): 69–88.
*"Endocrine Disrupting Chemicals and Women's Health Outcomes." NIH Guide, vol. 24, no. 38 (October 27, 1995) National Institute of Environmental Health Sciences Office of Research on Women's Health.
*"Facts About Environment-Related Diseases and Health Risks," NIEHS Fact Sheet #10, *Women's Health* (August 1997).
*Fraser, L. "The RU486 you don't know." *Mirabella* (March 1999) :92.
*Golan, R. *Optimal Wellness. New York: Ballantine Books, 1995*
*Goodman, A. "Abnormal Genital Tract Bleeding." *Clinical Cornerstone* 3(1) (2000): 25–35.
*Hodgen, G.D. "Gonadotropin-releasing hormone agonists: emerging modification of treatment regimens." *Current Opinion in Obstetrics and Gynecology* 3(3) (June 1991): 352–357.
*Kettel, L.M. et al. "Clinical efficacy of the antiprogesterone RU486 in the treatment of endometriosis and uterine fibroids." *Human Reproduction* Suppl 1 (June 1994) :116–120.
*Komesaroff, P.A. et al "Effects of Wild Yam Extract on Menopausal Symptoms, Lipids and Sex Hormones in Healthy Menopausal Women." *Climacteric*, vol. 4, no. 2. (June 2001)

*Lark, S.M. *Fibroid Tumors & Endometriosis.* Berkeley, CA: Celestial Arts, 1993.

*Letter to author from Duane Alexander, M.D., Director, National Institute of Child Health and Human Development, via e-mail, 2/10/01.

*Love, S.M. et al. *Dr. Susan Love's Hormone Book.* New York: Times Books, 1997.

*McKinney, M. "Hormone May Spur Tumor Blood Vessel Growth." *International Journal of Cancer.* 92(2001): 469–473.

*"Menstruation, pregnancy and menopause spell trouble for teeth," Academy of General Dentistry, Consumer Information, *www.agd.org.*

*Miller, L.G. "Herbal medicinals: selected clinical considerations focusing on known or potential drug-herb interactions." *Archives of Internal Medicine* 158(1998): 200–221.

*"Q & A's from the Cornell University Program on Breast Cancer and Environmental Risk Factors in New York State," NIEHS Fact Sheet #10 3/1998. *www.cfe.cornell.edu/bcerf/Factsheet/General/fctsht10.estrog.t.*

*Raloff, J. "Does yo-yo dieting pose cancer threat?" Science News Online, 3/15/97.

*Rich, W.M. "Cancer of the Uterus," CancerLink, *www.personal.u-net.com/~njh/cuterus.html*

*Schwartz, S.M. "Etiology of Uterine Leiomyomata ('Fibroids')." *faculty.washington.edu/stevesch/ss_ul.htm*

*Stewart, E.A. et al. "Leiomyoma-related bleeding: a classic hypothesis updated for the molecular era." *Human Reproduction Update* vol. 2, no. 4 (1996): 295–306.

*World Wildlife Fund, "A Warning from Wildlife," *www.wwf.org/new/issues/endocrine,* 1996.

*Wright, J.V. "Comparative Measurements of Serum Estriol, Estradiol and Estrone in Non-Pregnant, Premenopausal Women: A Preliminary Investigation." *www.throne.com/altmedrev/fulltext/estriol 4-4.*

Week 3

*"Acetaminophen may lower estrogen level," *Fertility and Sterility* 70(1998): 371–373.

*"Alpha interferon," The Access Project, *www.aidsinfonyc.org.*

*Center for Uterine Fibroids, *www.fibroids.net*

*"Experimental Technique Uses Lasers to Shrink Uterine Fibroids," drkoop.com. 11/28/00.

*The Fibroid Embolization Center, *www.uhmc.com/fibroid.htm.*

*Hale, E. "Taming Menstrual Cramps." *FDA Consumer Magazine,* *www.fda.gov/bbs/topics/consumer/con00004.html.* 6/91.

*Hickling, L. "New Procedures Improve Outcome of Uterine Fibroid Removal." *drkoop.com* 4/7/00.

*Law, P. et al. "Magnetic resonance-guided percutaneous laser ablation of uterine fibroids," *Journal of Magnetic Resonance Imaging* 12(4) (October 2000): 565–570.

*Lipman, J.C. "Uterine Artery Embolization for the Treatment of Sympto-matic Uterine Fibroids: A Review." *Applied Radiology* 29(7) (2000): 15–20.

*"Radiating Tumors with Protons." *Health News* (October 2000): 6.

*Ravina, J. et al. "Arterial embolization of uterine myomata: results of 184 cases." Presentation at 10th Anniversary International Conference for the Society for Minimally Invasive Therapy. September 4, 1998; London, Eng-land. MITAT 7 (suppl) (1998): 26–27.

*"Remarkable and persistent shrinkage of uterine leiomyoma associated with interferon alfa treatment for hepatitis." *The Lancet* vol. 353, no. 9170, (June 19, 1999).

*Smith, S.J. "Uterine Fibroids Embolization." *American Family Physician*, www.aafp.org/afp/20000615/3601.html. 6/15/00.

*"Uterine Fibroids," NIH pub 0051, *www.nih.gov/nihcd/html/publications.html.*

*"Uterine Leiomyomata," *ACOG Educational Bulletin* no. 192 (May 1994).

*Vilos, G.A. et al. "Pregnancy outcome after laparoscopic electromyolysis," *Journal of the American Association of Gynecologic Laparoscopists* 5(3) (August 1998): 289–292.

Week 4

*Aguillar, M. et al. "Your Medical Records. How Correct? How Important? How Damaging? How to Correct Your Medical Records; Comments on Your Medical Records." Cancer Links, *www.cancerlynx.com/records.html.* 4/2/01.

*Bennett, R.L. "Getting Medical Records and Information," *Genetic Health*, *www.genetichealth.com.* 8/28/01.

*Boule, M. "One woman's winning fight against the establishment." *The Ore-gonian* (March 4, 2001). *www.oregonlive.com/living/index.ssf?/columnists/ oregonian/01/03/1c_11boule04.frame.*

*Orin, R.D. "Health Laws That Can Save You Money—or Your Life," *The Washington Post*, 19, 2001, p. HE10.

Month 2

*Bailey, S. "Happy Thoughts May Prolong Life." Associated Press, 5/7/01.

*Benedict, O. "Medicine's Neglected Spirit." *Science & Spirit* vol. 9, issue 3: 3

*Blakeslee, S. "Enthusiasm of Doctor Can Give Pill Extra Kick." *The New York Times* October 13, 1998.

*Blakeslee, S. "Placebo's Prove So Powerful Even Experts Are Surprised." *The New York Times* October 13, 1998.

*Bunk, S. "Mind-Body Research Matures." *The Scientist* 15[12] (June 11, 2001): 8.

*Chamberlain, C. "Despair's Double Whammy, Among Older People, Depression May Raise Cancer Risk." *abcnews.go.com/sections/living/ InYourHead/allinyourhead_22.html.*

*Domar, A.D. et al. *Healing Mind, Healthy Woman*. New York: Delta Books 1996.

*Domar, A.D. et al. "Healthy Woman: The Mind-Body Connection." Women's Health Interactive." *www.womens-health.com/discussion/chat/archive1.html*. 3/20/97.

*Elcombe, S. et al. "The psychological effects of laparoscopy on women with chronic pelvic pain." *Psychological Medication* 27(5) (Sept. 1997): 1041–1050.

*Ellwood, R. *Finding the Quiet Mind*. Wheaton, IL: Theosophical Publishing House, 1983.

*Gawain, S. *Creative Visualization*. New York: Bantam Books, 1978.

*Gordon, W.A. *The Quotable Writer*. New York: McGraw-Hill, 2000.

*Horn, C. et al. "7 Surefire Strategies for Stress." *Natural Health* (April 1999): 121.

*Kenney, J.W. et al. "Interactive Model of Women's Stressors, Personality Traits and Health Problems" *Journal of Advanced Nursing* 32(2000): 249–258.

*Koenig, H.G. et al. "Use of Hospital Services, Religious Attendance, and Religious Affiliation," *Southern Medical Journal* vol. 91, no. 10 (1998), 925–932.

*Kotulak, R. *Inside The Brain*. Kansas City: Andrews and McMeel.

*"Life? Or Theatre?" by Charlotte Salomon (1917–1943). *www.jewishmuseum.org*.

*Martin, A.A. et al. "The effects of hypnosis on the labor process and birth outcomes of pregnant adolescents." *Journal of Family Practice* 50(2001): 441–443.

*Morris, L.B. "Totalled Recall." *Allure* (June 2001): 110.

*Norton, A. "Diabetes or depression often go together: study." *Diabetes Care* 24(2001): 1069–1078.

*Norton, A. "Just thinking about work may trigger stress." Reuters Health/Yahoo, *dailynews.yahoo.com*. 3/14/01.

*Oliver, G. et al. "Stress and Food Choice: A Laboratory Study." *Psychosomatic Medicine* 62(2000): 853–865.

*Saddler, P. et al. "Inner Healing for Women with Uterine Fibroids." Sunspire Health, *www.voiceofwomen.com/sunspire/home.html*.

*Schorr, M. "Music during eye surgery lowers blood pressure." *Psychosomatic Medicine* 63(2001): 487–492.

*"Self-confidence can make childbirth less painful." *Journal of Psychosomatic Obstetrics and Gynecology*. 21(2000):219–224.

*"Stress and Cancer: Mind, Body, and Immunity." *Women's Health Advocate* 5(8) (November 1998): 40.

*"Survey of the American Public, HMO Professionals and Family Physicians Determine General Attitudes Toward Spirituality as a Component of the Healing Process." 1998 Yankelovich survey.

*Van Biema, D. "A Test of the Healing Power of Prayer." *Time* 152(15) (October 12, 1998): 72.

*"Women: Taking the Stress Home," *Mind/Body Health* newsletter vol. VIII, no. 3 (1999): 5.

Month 3

*"Acupuncture and Chinese Medicine in Women's Health:" SHN Chat Room Transcript, *www.shn.net/cgi-bin*.

*"Alternative Medicine—The Risks of Untested and Unregulated Remedies." *The New England Journal of Medicine* vol. 339, no. 12 (September 17, 1998):

*Angelo, J. *Hands-On Healing*. Rochester, VT: Healing Arts Press, 1994.

*Associated Press. "Study: Supplements Need New Rules," *The New York Times, www.nytimes.com*. 4/18/01.

*Brody, J.E. "Americans Gamble on Herbs as Medicine," *The New York Times*, 9 February 1999.

*Cardoso, S.H. Center for Biomedical Informatics State University of Campinas, Brazil, *www.epub.org.br/cm/n03/mente/hormones_I.htm*.

*Cole, J. "News from the Sex Labs, Let's Get Personal." *Health* (September 2000): 176.

*Cummings, S. et al. *Everybody's Guide to Homeopathic Medicine*. New York: Tarcher/Putnam 1997.

*Cutler, W.B. *Hysterectomy: Before and After*. HarperPerennial 1988.

*Dwass, E. "Vagina Monologues Has Doctors Listening." *USA Today www.usatoday.com* 6/19/2001.

*"Dysmenorrhea (Menstrual Pain)." Alternative Medicine, Thrive Online, *thriveonline.oxygen.com*.

*Epstein, R.H. "Major Medical Mystery: Why People Avoid Doctors." *The New York Times*, 31 October 2000.

*Fackelmann, K. "Researchers study herbal remedies for hot flashes." Science News Online, 6/20/98; *Science News* vol. 153, no. 25 (June 20, 1998): 392.

*Fox, C.A. "Some aspects and implications of coital physiology." *Journal of Sex and Marital Therapy* 2(3) (Fall 1976): 205–213.

*Gardner, M.B., "Facts About Oral Contraceptives," Office of Research Reporting, National Institute of Child Health and Human Development (NICHD), 1983.

*Gilkeson, J. *Energy Healing: A Pathway to Inner Growth*. New York: Marlowe & Co., 2000.

*Goldfarb, H.A. et al. *The No-Hysterectomy Option: Your Body—Your Choice*. New York: John Wiley & Sons, 1997.

*Goldstein, S.R. et al. *The Estrogen Alternative*. New York: G.P. Putnam's Sons, 1998.

*Grady, D. "To Aid Doctors, A.M.A. Journal Devotes Entire Issue to Alternative Medicine." *The New York Times*, 11 November 1998.

*Graedon, J. et al. *The People's Pharmacy*. New York: St. Martin's Griffin, 2001.

*"Gynecological Herbs," *clinical.caregroup.org.*

*Hampton, S. "The Human Sexual Response Cycle." *www.umkc.edu/sites/hsw/Sexresponse/Index.html.*

*Harrar, S. et al. *Women's Healing Herbs.* Emmaus, PA: Rodale Press 1999.

*Hasson, H.M. "Cervical removal at hysterectomy for benign disease. Risks and benefits." *Journal of Reproductive Medicine* 38(10) (October 1993): 781–790.

*Hobbs, C. "Vitex, The Hormone Balancing Herb." Health World Online.

Greaterchinaherbs.lycosasia.com/my/english/l5i6.html.

*"Kampo Therapy and Clinical Research Put Down Roots in Germany." Kampo Today vol. 3, no. 2 (March 1999) *www.tsumura.co.jp.*

*Lee, Y. "Acupuncture It's More Than Just Needles." The National Council on Women's Health *www.womens-health.com/affiliations/affiliates/ncwh/news/fall96/fa96_a5.html.*

*Loeliger, W. "Complementary Medicine: Acupuncture Part II." GBMC Alternative and Complementary Health Center *www.wrc-gbmc.org/Library.*

*Lonsdorf, N. *A Woman's Best Medicine.* New York: Tarcher/Putnam, 1995.

*Love, S.M. et al. *Dr. Susan Love's Hormone Book,* New York: Times Books, 1997.

*Martin, R.W. "Tumors, Cysts, Fibroids, Cancer: Is Your Wood Overgrown?" AltMed Health Channel, AOL.

*McGregor, D.K. *From Midwives to Medicine.* Piscataway, NJ: Rutgers University Press 1998.

*McIntyre, A. *The Complete Woman's Herbal.* New York: Henry Holt, 1995.

*Mehl-Madrona, L. "Complementary Medicine Treatment of Uterine Fibroids." Center for Complementary Medicine, University of Pittsburgh Medical Center.

*Mundell, E.J. "Bacteria, fungi found in herbal meds: study," Reuters, 5/23/2001.

*Nissim, R. *Natural Healing in Gynaecology.* Pandora, 1996.

*Null, G. *The Woman's Encyclopedia of Natural Healing.* Seven Stories Press, 1996.

*Pettit, J.L. "Alternative Medicine—Black Cohosh." *Clinician Reviews* 10(4) (2000): 117–118, 121.

*"Recommendations for fibroids treatment using TCM." Healthsky.com, *www.healthsky.com.*

*Reichenberg-Ullman, J. "Healing Uterine Fibroids." Healthy Net, *www.healthy.net.*

*Reichenberg-Ullman, J. "What do I need to know about homeopathic treatment?" Healthy Net, *www.healthy.net.*

*"Report: Herbal Remedies Cause Problems in Surgery." Reuters, July 10 2001.

*Rister, R. "Kampo Medicine." *www.letsliveonline.com.*

*Sakamoto, S. et al. "Conservative management for perimenopausal women with uterine leiomyomas using Chinese herbal medicines and synthetic analogs of gonadotrophin-releasing hormone." *In Vivo* 12(3) (May-June 1998): 333–337.

*"Shakuyaku-kanzo-to's Efficacy For Acute Muscle Spasm Validated by Clinical Studies, Basic Research." *Kampo Today* vol. 4, no. 1 (April 2000).

*Stolberg, S.G. "The Estrogen Alternative." *The New York Times Magazine* *www.nytimes.com*. 5/16/2001.

*"Traditional Chinese Medicine," Body Mind Wellness Center, *www.bodymindwellnesscenter.com*.

*Ullman, D. *The Consumer's Guide to Homeopathy*. New York: Tarcher/Putnam, 1996.

*Varnell, M.A. "Herbs Used for Menopause Act Like Estrogen." *cancerpage.com*, 6/14/2000.

*Villoldo, A. *Shaman, Healer, Sage*. New York: Harmony Books, 2000.

*Vukovic, L. "Home Remedies." *Natural Health* (April 1999): 140.

*Weil, A. "Acupuncture, New Uses for an Ancient Art." *Dr. Andrew Weil's Self Healing*, 4/98:2.

*Weston, L.C. " ⟨handwritten: ? 1998⟩ n Sexuality." ONHEALTH ⟨handwritten: Have newer titles. + 1 in Cart⟩ 5017.asp. 9/17/98.

*Woodham, A. e s. Dorling Kindersley, 1997.

*Woods, T. "The nd and Third Chakras." AltN

*Yan, H. et al. "[T eated with acupuncture]." *Zhen C*

*Zand, J. "Herbal thWorld Online.

*Zhou, J. et al. "[C⟨...⟩al and experimental study on improving cellular immunological function of uterine myoma patients by xiaoliu tablet]." *Zhongguo Zhong Xi Yi Jie He Za Zhi* 17(5) (May 1997): 277–279.

Month 4

*"Acetaminophen may lower estrogen level." *Fertility and Sterility* 70(1998): 371–373.

*Adashi, E.Y. "Long-term gonadotropin-releasing hormone agonist therapy: the evolving issue of steroidal "add-back" paradigms." *Keio Journal of Medicine* 44(4) (December 1995): 124–132.

*Agency for Healthcare Research and Quality. *Management of Uterine Fibroids*. Summary, Evidence Report/Technology Assessment: Number 34. AHRQ Publication No. 01-E051, January 2001.

*Alfini, P. et al. "Treatment of uterine fibroma with goserelin [Trattamento del fibroma uterino con Goserelin]." *Annali di Ostettricia, Ginecologia, Medicine Perinatale* 112(6) (November–December 1991): 359–367.

*Auber, G. et al. "Use of GnRH depot analogue in the treatment of uterine fibroids." *Acta Europaea Fertilitatis* 21(4) (July–August 1990): 185–189.

*Broder, M.S. et al. "Uterine Artery Embolization: A Systematic Review of the Literature and Proposal for Research." The Rand Corp., p. 4.

*Center for Uterine Fibroids , *www.fibroids.net*.

*Cagnacci, A. et al. "Role of goserelin-depot in the clinical management of uterine fibroids." *Clinical and Experimental Obstetrics and Gynaecology* 21(4) (1994): 263–265.

*Chipato, T. et al. "Pelvic pain complicating LHRH analogue treatment of fibroids." *Australia and New Zealand Journal of Obstetrics and Gynaecology* 31(4) (November 1991): 383–384.

*Chrisp, P. et al. "Goserelin. A review of its pharmacodynamic and pharma- cokinetic properties, and clinical use in sex hormone-related conditions." *Drugs* 41(2) (February 1991): 254–288.

*Christiansen, J.K. "The facts about fibroids. Presentation and latest manage- ment options." *Postgraduate Medicine* 94(3) (September 1993): 129–134, 137.

*Conn, P.M. and W.F. Crowley, Jr. "Gonadotropin-releasing hormone and its analogs," *Annual Review of Medicine* 45(1994): 391–405.

*Crosignani, P.G. et al. "GnRH agonists before surgery for uterine leiomy- omas." *Journal of Reproductive Medicine* 41(6) (June 1996): 415–421.

*Eldar-Geva, T. et al. "Effect of intramural, subserosal, and submucosal uter- ine fibroids on the outcome of assisted reproductive technology treat- ment." *Fertility and Sterility* 70(4) (October 1998): 687–691.

*Estrace Prescription Information, *www.rxmed.com/monographs/estrace.html*, rxmed website.

*"Estrogens and Progestins Oral Contraceptives (Systemic)." National Library of Medicine, *www.nih.org*. 1/24/01.

*The Fibroid Embolization Center, *www.uhmc.com/fibroid.htm*.

*Furui, T. "Differential efficacy of gonadotropin-releasing hormone (GnRH) agonist treatment on pedunculated and degenerated myomas: a retrospec- tive study of 630 women." *Journal of Obstetrics & Gynecology*. vol. 20, no. 5 (September 2000): 504–506.

*Gaby, A.R. The Natural Hormone Alternative, *www.voiceofwomen.com/arti- cles/naturalhormones.html*.

*Gardner, R.L. et al. "Cornual fibroids: a conservative approach to restoring tubal patency using a gonadotropin-releasing hormone agonist (goserelin) with successful pregnancy." *Fertility and Sterility* 52(2) (August 1989): 332–334.

*Garner, C. "Uses of GnRH agonists." *Journal of Obstetric, Gynecologic, and Neonatal Nursing* 23(7) (September 1994): 563–570.

*Ginsburg, J. et al. "Clinical experience with tibolone (Livial) over 8 years." Maturitas 21(1) (January 1995): 71–76.

*Givens, M. et al. "Fibroids," e Medicine Consumer Journal, May 31 2001, Vol. 2, No.5.

*Golan, A. "GnRH analogues in the treatment of uterine fibroids." *Human Reproduction* 11 Suppl 3 (November 1996): 33–41.

*Golan, A. et al. "Pre-operative gonadotrophin-releasing hormone agonist treatment in surgery for uterine leiomyomata." *Human Reproduction* 8(3) (March 1993): 450–452.

*Greene, H. "Understanding Off-Label Drug Usage." *HealthNews* (March 2001): 4.

*Hale, E. "Taming Menstrual Cramps." *FDA Consumer Magazine*
  www.fda.gov/bbs/topics/consumer/con0004.html. 6/91.
*Henig, R.M. "Behind the Buzz on Designer Estrogens." *The New York Times*
  6/21/98: WH4.
*Hurkainen, R. et al. "Early Report: Quality of Life and Cost-effectiveness of
  Levonorgestrel-releasing Intrauterine System versus Hysterectomy for
  Treatment of Menorrhagia: a randomized trial." *The Lancet* 357(2001):
  273–277.
*Kettel, L.M. et al. "Clinical efficacy of the antiprogesterone RU486 in the
  treatment of endometriosis and uterine fibroids." *Human Reproduction* 9
  Suppl 1 (June 1994): 116–120.
*Kuhlmann, M. et al. "Uterine leiomyomata and sterility: therapy with
  gonadotropin-releasing hormone agonists and leiomyomectomy." *Gynecol-
  ogy and Endocrinology* 11(3) (June 1997): 169–174.
*Lewin, T. "Pending F.D.A. Approval, French Abortion Pill is Getting Limited
  Use Here," *The New York Times*, 5 March 2000.
*Lipman, J.C. "Uterine Artery Embolization for the Treatment of Sympto-
  matic Uterine Fibroids: A Review." *Applied Radiology* 29(7): 15–20.
*Love, S.M. et al. *Dr. Susan Love's Hormone Book,* Times Books, 1997.
*Mayfield, E. "Choosing a Treatment for Uterine Fibroids." *FDA Consumer
  Magazine* (October 15, 1997).
*McKinney, M. "Osteoporosis Drug Found to Shrink Uterine Fibroids." *Fer-
  tility and Sterility* 76(2001): 38–43.
*Nelson, A. "Contraceptive Update Y2K: Need for Contraceptive and New
  Contraceptive Options." *Clinical Cornerstone* 3(1) (2000): 48–62.
*Nencioni, T. et al. "Gonadotropin releasing hormone agonist therapy and its
  effect on bone mass," *Gynecology and Endocrinology* 5(1) (March 1991):
  45–56.
*"Oral contraceptive use and benign gynecological conditions. A review."
  Contraception 57(1) (January 1998): 11–18.
*Ortho Pharmaceuticals, OrthoNorethindrone-Ethinyl EstradiolOral Contra-
  ceptive, *www.rxmed.com/monographs/orthotab.html.*
*"An Overview of Pill Formulations." *Clinical Proceedings* Electronic Edition.
  www.arhp.org/clinical/mar99c.htm.
*Perry, C.M. et al. "Goserelin. A review of its pharmacodynamic and pharma-
  cokinetic properties, and therapeutic use in benign gynaecological disorders." *Drugs* 51(2) (February 1996): 319–346.
*Rako, S. "Testosterone supplemental therapy after hysterectomy with or
  without concomitant oophorectomy: estrogen alone is not enough." *Journal of Women's Health and Gender Based Medicine* 9(8) (October
  2000):917–923.
*Reinsch, R.C. et al. "The effects of RU 486 and leuprolide acetate on uter-
  ine artery blood flow in the fibroid uterus: a prospective, randomized
  study." *American Journal of Obstetrics and Gynecology* 170(6) (June 1994):
  1623–1628.

*Schwartz, L.B. et al. "Does the Use of Postmenopausal Hormone Replacement Therapy Influence the Size of Uterine Leiomyomata? A Preliminary Report." *Menopause* (Spring 1996): 38–43.

*Starczewski, A. et al. "Intrauterine therapy with levonorgestrel releasing IUD of women with hypermenorrhea secondary to uterine fibroids." *Ginekologia Polska* 71(9) (September 2000): 1221–1225.

*Stjernquist, M. "Treatment of uterine fibroids with GnRH-analogues prior to hysterectomy." *Acta Obstetricia et Gynecologica Scandinavica* 164 Suppl (1997): 94–97.

*Sutton, C.J.G. "Treatment of large uterine fibroids." *British Journal of Obstetrics and Gynaecology* 103(1996):494–496.

*Thorneycroft, I.A. et al. "Ultra-Low-Dose Contraceptives: Are They Right for Your Patient?" Medscape Women's Health 6(4) (July 3, 2001).

*"Uterine Fibroids," NIH pub 0051, *www.nih.gov/nichd/html/publications.html.*

*"Uterine Leiomyomata," *ACOG Educational Bulletin* no. 192 (May 1994).

*van Leusden, H.A. "Symptom-free interval after triptorelin treatment of uterine fibroids: long-term results." *Gynecological Endocrinology* 6(3) (September 1992): 189–198.

*Voelker, R. "Advisory on Contraceptives." *JAMA* vol. 284 no. 8 (August 23/30, 2000): 951.

*Williams, I.A. et al. "Effect of nafarelin on uterine fibroids measured by ultrasound and magnetic resonance imaging." *European Journal of Obstetrics, Gynecology, and Reproductive Biology* 1990 34(1-2) (January–February 1990): 111–117.

*Wright, J.V. et al. "Comparative Measurements of Serum Estriol, Estradiol, and Estrone in Non-pregnant, Premenopausal Women: A Preliminary Investigation." *Alternative Medicine Review* vol. 4, no. 4 *www.thorne.com/altmedrev/fulltext/estriol44.html.* 8/99.

*Yang, Y et al. "Treatment of uterine leiomyoma by two different doses of mifepristone." *Chung Hua Fu Chan Ko Tsa Chih* 31(10) (October 1996): 624–626.

Month 5

*Agency for Healthcare Research and Quality. *Management of Uterine Fibroids.* Summary, Evidence Report/Technology Assessment: Number 34. AHRQ Publication No. 01-E051 (January 2001).

*Brown, D. et al. "Caesarean myomectomy—a safe procedure. A retrospective case controlled study." *Journal of Obstetrics and Gynecology* vol. 19 no. 2 (March 1999).

*Chan, P.D. et al. *Current Clinical Strategies Gynecology and Obstetrics.* Current Clinical Strategies Publishing (1997 Edition) www.CCSPublishing.com: #107, #122.

*Chopelas, A. "Fibroid Study and Research Program: Causes, Symptoms, Relief and Possible Solutions." 1997, originally published on Intradesign.com.

*Coronado, G.D. et al. "Complications in pregnancy, labor, and delivery with uterine leiomyomas: a population-based study." *Obstetrics and Gynecology* 95(5) (May 2000): 764–769.

*Curtis, G.B. *Your Pregnancy Questions & Answers*. Tucson: Fisher Books, 1995.

*Dietterich, C. et al. "The presence of small uterine fibroids not distorting the endometrial cavity does not adversely affect conception outcome following embryo transfer in older recipients." *Clinical and Experimental Obstetrics and Gynecology* 27(3-4) (2000): 168–170.

*Dildy, G.A. et al. "Indomethacin for the treatment of symptomatic leiomyoma uteri during pregnancy." *American Journal of Perinatology* 9(3) (May 1992): 185–189.

*Eldar-Geva, T. et al. "Effect of intramural, subserosal, and submucosal uterine fibroids on the outcome of assisted reproductive technology treatment." *Fertility and Sterility* 70(4) (October 1998): 687–691.

*Eisenberg, A. et al. *What to Expect When You're Expecting*. New York: Workman Publishing, 1991.

*The Fibroid Embolization Center, *www.uhmc.com/fibroid.htm*.

*Friedman, L. et al. *A Woman Doctor's Guide to Miscarriage*. New York: Hyperion, 1996.

*Goodman, R.M. *Planning for a Healthy Baby: A Guide to Genetic and Environmental Risks*, New York: Oxford University Press, 1986.

*Hales, D. et al. *Intensive Caring: New Hope for High-Risk Pregnancy*. New York: Crown Publishers, Inc., 1990.

*Hasan, F. et al. "Uterine leiomyomata in pregnancy." *International Journal of Gynecology & Obstetrics*. 34(1) (January 1991): 45–48.

*Hatcher, R. et al. "Infertility Evaluation." ThriveOnline.com.

*Hutcherson, H. et al. *Having Your Baby: A Guide for African-American Women*. New York: One World/Ballantine Books, 1997.

*Jun, S.H. et al. "Uterine leiomyomas and their effect on in vitro fertilization outcome: a retrospective study." *Journal of Assisted Reproduction and Genetics* 18(3) (March 2001): 139–143.

*Katz, et al. "Complications of uterine leiomyomas in pregnancy." *Obstetrics and Gynecology* 73(4) (1989): 593–596.

*Lark, S. *Fibroid Tumors & Endometriosis Self Help Book*. Berkeley, CA: Celestial Arts, 1995.

*Larson, D.E. *The Mayo Clinic Family Health Book*. New York: William Morrow & Co., 1996.

*Maderas, L. *Womancare*. New York: Avon Books, 1984.

*Siccardi, D.C. "Leiomyomas." *Obstetrics & Gynecology*, Medstudents, www.medstudents.com/br/ginob/ginob6.htm.

*Slupik, R.I. *American Medical Association Complete Guide to Women's Health*. New York: Random House, 1996.

*Sudik, R. et al. "Fertility and pregnancy outcome after myomectomy in sterility patients." *European Journal of Obstetrics, Gynecology, and Reproductive Biology* 65(2) (April 1996): 209–214.

*"Uterine Leiomyomata." *ACOG Educational Bulletin* no. 192, (May 1994).

Month 6

*Atlanta Reproductive Health Center. "A Couple's Guide to Hysterosalpin-gogram [HSG]." *www.ivf.com/hsg.ht.*

*Center for Uterine Fibroids, *www.fibroids.net.*

*Feste, J. "Preoperative Evaluation—Medical Treatment of Uterine Fibroids." GynEndoscopy.com.

*Goldberg, J.M. et al. "Gasless Gynecologic Laparoscopy: A Work in Progress." *The Female Patient* (Feb. 1998).

*Goldfarb, H.A. et al. *The No-Hysterectomy Option: Your Body—Your Choice.* New York: John Wiley & Sons, 1997.

*Goodman, A. "Abnormal Genital Tract Bleeding." *Clinical Cornerstone* 3(1) (2000): 25–35.

*Griffith, H.W. *Complete Guide to Medical Tests* (see p. 19 for rest of info).

*Griffith, H.W. *Complete Guide to Symptoms, Illness & Surgery.* New York: The Putnam Book Group Inc., 1995. *www.thriveonline.com/health/Library/medtests/medtest221.ht.*

*Kirby, D. "Patients Embrace New Generation of Imaging Machines." *The New York Times, www.nytimes.com.* 5/8/01.

*Lauersen, N. et al. *It's Your Body.* New York: Berkley Books, 1977.

*"Lidocaine Spray Reduces Pain," *Fertility and Sterility* 1998; 69: 549-551

*Lipman, J.C. "Uterine Artery Embolization for the Treatment of Symptomatic Uterine Fibroids: A Review." *Applied Radiology* 29(7) (2000): 15–20.

*"MR Safety." *kanal.arad.upmc.edu/safety/psychological.html.*

*Northrup, C. *Women's Bodies, Women's Wisdom.* New York: Bantam Books, 1994.

*Perloe, M. et al. "Miracle Babies and Other Happy Endings for Couples With Fertility Problems." Atlanta Reproductive Health Center, *www.ivf.com/ch16mb.ht.* 1986.

*Sobel, D.S. et al. *The Healthy Mind, Healthy Body Handbook.* Patient Education Media, Inc., 1996.

*Spaner, S.J. et al. "A Brief History of Endoscopy, Laparoscopy, and Laparoscopic Surgery." *Journal of Laparoendoscopy,* Advanced Surgical Techniques. (Dec. 1997): 369–373.

Month 7

*Agency for Healthcare Research and Quality. *Management of Uterine Fibroids.* Summary. Evidence Report/Technology Assessment: 34. AHRQ Publication No. 01-E051, (January 2001).

*American Cancer Society. "New Blood Test for Ovarian Cancer Shows Promise." *www2.cancer.org/zine/002_10081998_0.html;* and *www.cancer.org/statistics/cff98/selectedcancers.html.*

*Botsis, D. et al. "Endometrial Thickness and Doppler Velocimetry in Women with Peri- and Postmenopausal Bleeding, before Endometrial Sampling." *European Menopause Journal* 3(2) (1996): 42–46.

*Braun, R.D. "Laminaria Tents." *www.obgyn.net*.

*Bruchak, K.T. "CA125 (Cancer Antigen 125)." University of Pennsylvania Cancer Center, Posted Date: February 21, 1997.

*Carlson, K.J. et al. "Indications for hysterectomy." *The New England Journal of Medicine* 328(12) (1993): 856–860.

*Center for Uterine Fibroids, *www.fibroids.net*.

*"Common Uterine Conditions: Options for Treatment." AHCPR Publication No. 98-0003, (Dec. 1997). Agency for Health Care Policy and Research. *www.ahcpr.gov/consumer/uterine1.htm*.

*"Disorders of the Uterus: Leiomyomata Uteri." *Journal of Obstetrics & Gynecology*. (August 1998).

*Dover, R.W. et al. "Sarcomas and the conservative management of uterine fibroids: a cause for concern?" *Australia and New Zealand Journal of Obstetrics and Gynecology* 40(3) (August 2000): 308–312.

*Dwass, E. "Vagina Monologues has doctors listening," *USA Today*, 19 June 2001, *www.usatoday.com*.

*Epstein, R.H. "Major Medical Mystery: Why People Avoid Doctors." *The New York Times*, 31 October 2000.

*Ferrini, R. "Screening Asymptomatic Women for Ovarian Cancer, American College of Preventive Medicine Practice Policy." *American Journal of Preventive Medicine* 13(6) (November/December 1997): 444–446.

*Feste, J. "Medical Treatment of Uterine Fibroids." Gyn-Endoscopy.com.

*"Genetic Test May Act As 'Second Opinion' For Women Facing Hysterectomies." Doctors Guide Website, *www.pslgroup.co/dg/2ef6e.htm*.

*Jacobs, I. et al. "Is Serum CA-125 a Useful Screening Test for Ovarian Cancer? Paper: Risk of Diagnosis of Ovarian Cancer after Raised Serum CA-125 Concentration: A Prospective Cohort Study." *BMJ* 313(1996): 1355–1358.

*Laurensen, N. et al. *It's Your Body: A Woman's Guide to Gynecology*. New York: Berkley Books, 1982.

*"Looking Inside the Uterus." *Harvard Women's Health Watch*. (January 1997): 4–5.

*National Cancer Institute, "What You Need to Know About Cancer of the Uterus," National Institutes of Health: 4.

Pear, R. "Incompetent Physicians Are Rarely Reported as Law Requires," *The New York Times*, 29 May 2001.

*"Primary Care Physicians' Experience of Financial Incentives in Managed-Care Systems." *The New England Journal of Medicine*. vol. 339, no. 21 (November 19, 1998). *www.nejm.org/content/1998/0339/0021/1516.asp*.

*Rich, W.M. "Cancer of the Uterus." CancerLink, *www.personal.u-net.com/~njh/cuterus.html*.

*Rostler, S. "U.S. Women Prefer Female Ob/Gyns: Survey." Reuters Health, *dailynews.yahoo.com*. 5/1/2001.

*Siccardi, D.C. "Leiomyomas," *Obstetrics & Gynecology*, Medstudents, *www.medstudents.com.br/ginob/ginob6.htm*

*"Uterine Fibroids." National Institutes of Health, *www.nih.gov/nichd/html/news/uterine.htm*.

*"Uterine Leiomyomata." *ACOG Educational Bulletin* Number 192, (May 1994).

*"Uterine Sarcoma," NCI/PDQ Patient Statement, OncoLink, pdq@oncolink.upenn.edu.

*"VersaPoint System for Fibroid Removal Cleared by FDA." Menlo Park, CA, PConsulting group Inc., *www.pslgroup.com*. 11/4/96.

*Weinstein, K. *Living With Endometriosis*. Reading, MA: Addison-Wesley Publishing Co., 1987.

*"Women's Health Facts and Links." Society for Women's Health Research, *www.womens-health.org*. 6/13/01.

Month 8

*Agency for Health Care Policy and Research. *Common Uterine Conditions: Options for Treatment*. AHCPR Publication No. 98-0003, (December 1997). *www.ahcpr.gov/consumer/uterine1.htm*.

*Agency for Healthcare Research and Quality. *Management of Uterine Fibroids*. Summary, Evidence Report/Technology Assessment: Number 34. AHRQ Publication No. 01-E051, (January 2001). *www.ahrq.gov/clinic/utersumm.htm*.

*Kjerulff, K.H. et al. "Hysterectomy and Race." *Obstetrics and Gynecology* 82(5) (November 1993): 757–764.

*Kjerulff, K.H. et al. "The Socioeconomic Correlates of Hysterectomies in the United States." *American Journal of Public Health* 1993; 83(1) (1993): 106–108.

*Lilford, R. "Hysterectomy: Will It Pay the Bills in 2007?" *BMJ* 314 (1997): 160.

*Marshall, D. "Snip Judgements." *Mirabella* 6(4) (September 1994): 212–215.

*Mayfield, E. "Choosing a Treatment for Uterine Fibroids." *FDA Consumer Magazine* (October 15, 2001).

*"The Miracle of Endoscopy." *To Your Health*, Stanford University Hospital (summer 1993): 4–5.

*Settnes, A. et al. "Hysterectomy in a Danish cohort. Prevalence, incidence and socio-demographic characteristics." *Acta Obstetricia et Gynecologica Scandinavica* 75(3) (March 1996): 274–280.

*Subramanian, S. et al. "Uterine artery embolization for leiomyomata: resource use and cost estimation." *Journal of Vascular and Interventional Radiology* 12(5) (May): 571–574.

*West, S. *The Hysterectomy Hoax*. New York: Main Street Books, Doubleday, 1994.

Month 9

*Amato, P. et al. "Transient ovarian failure: a complication of uterine artery embolization." *Fertility and Sterility* 75(2) (February 2001): 438–439.

*Andersen, P.E. et al. "Uterine artery embolization of symptomatic uterine fibroids; Initial success and short-term results." *Acta Radiologica* 42(2) (March 2001): 234–238.

*Associated Press, "Lasers Help Shrink Uterine Fibroid Tumors," *The New York Times*, 12 December 2000.

*Berkowitz, R.P. et al. "Vaginal expulsion of submucosal fibroids after uterine artery embolization. A report of three cases." *Journal of Reproductive Medicine*. 44(4) (April 1999): 373–376.

*Brunereau, L. et al. "Uterine artery embolization in the primary treatment of uterine leiomyomas: technical features and prospective follow-up with clinical and sonographic examinations in 58 patients." *American Journal of Roentgenology* 175(5) (November 2000): 1267–1272.

*DeNoon, D.J. "Outpatient Fibroid Treatment Beats Open Surgery." WebMD Medical News, 3/6/01.

*Donnez, J. et al. "Review." *Human Reproduction Update*, 6(6) (November-December 2000): 609–613.

*Downie, A.C. et al. "Bilateral uterine artery embolisation to treat uterine fibroids: Initial experience." *Cardiovascular Interventional Radiology* 21(suppl):142:357–360, 1998.

*Dover, R.W. et al. "Uterine artery embolisation for symptomatic fibroids." *Medical Journal of Australia* 172(5) (March 6, 2000): 233–236.

*Greenberg, M.D. et al. "Medical and socioeconomic impact of uterine fibroids." *Obstetrics and Gynecology Clinics of North America* 22(1995): 625–636.

*Hickling, L. "New Procedures Improve Outcome of Uterine Fibroid Removal." *drkoop.com*, 4/7/00.

*Hutchins, F.L. "Abdominal myomectomy as a treatment for symptomatic uterine fibroids," *Obstetrics and Gynecology Clinics of North America* 22(1995): 781–789.

*LaMorte, A.I. et al. "Morbidity associated with abdominal myomectomy." *Obstetrics and Gynecology* 82 (1993): 897–900.

*Law, P. et al. "Magnetic-resonance guided percutaneous laser ablation of uterine fibroids." *The Lancet* vol. 354, no. 9195 (December 11, 1999).

*Levie, M. "Uterine Artery Embolization: Laparoscopic Myomectomy." XVI World Congress of the International Federation of Gynecology and Obstetrics, Women's Health Conference Summaries, Medscape 2000.

*Lipman, J.C. "Uterine Artery Embolization for the Treatment of Symptomatic Uterine Fibroids: A Review." *Applied Radiology* 29(7) (2000): 15–20.

*McLucas, B. et al. "Uterine fibroid embolization: nonsurgical treatment for symptomatic fibroids." *Journal of the American College of Surgeons* 192(1) (January 2001): 95–105.

*Pelage, J.P. et al. "Fibroid-related menorrhagia: Treatment with superselective embolization of the uterine arteries and midterm follow-up." *Radiology* 215 (2000): 428–431.

*Pollard, R.R. et al. "Prolapsed cervical myoma after uterine artery emboliza-
tion. A case report." *Journal of Reproductive Medicine* 46(5) (May 2001):
499–500.

*Ravina, J. et al. "Arterial embolisation to treat uterine myomata." *The Lancet*
346 (1995): 671–672.

*Roberts, P.D. "Uterine Artery Embolization as a Treatment for Uterine
Fibroids: Literature Review." *www.proberts.net.* 5/2/01.

*Roth, A.R. et al. "Pain after uterine artery embolization for leiomyomata: can
its severity be predicted and does severity predict outcome?" *Journal of
Vascular and Interventional Radiology* 11(8) (September 2000):
1047–1052.

*SCVIR survey 1999: Preparatory brief for FDA Obstetrics & Gynecology
Devices Panel, *SCVIR News*, Fairfax, VA, vol. 12, no. 6 (November/
December, 1999).

*Spies, J.B. et al. "Uterine fibroid embolization: measurement of health-
related quality of life before and after therapy." *Journal of Vascular and
Interventional Radiology* 10(10) (November-December 1999): 1293–1303.

*Smith, S.J. "Uterine Fibroid Embolization," *American Family Physician*
www.aafp.org/afp/20000615/3601.html. 6/15/00.

*Vedantham, S. et al. "Uterine Artery Embolization for Fibroids: Considera-
tions in Patient Selection and Clinical Follow-up." Medscape Women's
Health 4(5) (1999) *www.medscape.com/Medscape/WomensHealth/
journal/1999/v04.n05.*

*Vilos, G.A. et al. "Pregnancy outcome after laparoscopic electromyolysis."
Journal of the American Association of Gynecology Laparoscopists 5(3)
(August 1998): 289–292.

*Wong, G.C. et al. "Uterine artery embolization: a minimally invasive tech-
nique for the treatment of uterine fibroids." *Journal of Women's Health and
Gender Based Medicine* 9(4) (May 2000): 357–362.

*Worthington-Kirsch, R.L. et al. "Uterine arterial embolization for the man-
agement of leiomyomas: quality-of-life assessment and clinical response."
Radiology 208 (1998): 625–629.

Month 10

*Agency for Healthcare Research and Quality. *Management of Uterine
Fibroids*. Summary, Evidence Report/Technology Assessment: Number 34.
AHRQ Publication No. 01-E051, January 2001.

*Babaknia, A. et al. "Pregnancy success following abdominal myomectomy
for infertility." *Fertility and Sterility* 30(6) (December 1978): 644–647.

*Berger, G.S. "Outpatient Uterine Myomectomy." INCIID Home, InterNa-
tional Council on Infertility Information Dissemination,
www.inciid.org/reproductive-surgery.html.

*"Breakthrough Technology Reduces Post-Surgical Complications."
www.pslgroup.com/dg/2D082.htm. 6/23/97.

*Broder, M.S. et al. "Uterine Artery Embolization: A Systematic Review of
the Literature and Proposal for Research." The Rand Corp: 5, 21.

*Books, P.G. "Resectoscopic Myoma Vaporizer." *The Journal of Reproductive Medicine* vol. 40, no. 11 (November 1995): 791–795.

*Candiani, G.B. et al. "Risk of recurrence after myomectomy." *British Journal of Obstetrics and Gynaecology* 98(1991): 385–389.

*Center for Uterine Fibroids, *www.fibroids.net*.

*Darai, E. et al. "Fertility after laparoscopic myomectomy: preliminary results." *Human Reproduction* 12(9) (September 1997): 1931–1934.

*Emanuel, M.H. et al. Long-term results of hysteroscopic myomectomy for abnormal uterine bleeding." *Obstetrics and Gynecology* 93(5 Pt 1) (May 1999): 743–748.

*Fedele, L. et al. "Recurrence of fibroids after myomectomy: A transvaginal study." *Human Reproduction* 10 (1995): 1795–1796.

*Feste, J. "Endometrial Ablation Rectoscope/Myomectomy Techniques and Complications." *www.obgyn.net/ah/articles/ablrecfib/ablrecfib.htm*.

*The Fibroid Embolization Center, *www.uhmc.com/fibroid.htm*.

*Friedman, L. et al. *A Woman Doctor's Guide to Miscarriage*. New York: Hyperion, 1996.

*Galen, D.I. et al. "Outpatient Laparoscopic Hysterectomy: A Review of 50 Patients." *Journal of the American Association of Gynecologic Laparoscopists* vol. 1, no. 3 (May 1994).

*Goldfarb, H.A. et al. *The No-Hysterectomy Option: Your Body—Your Choice*. New York: John Wiley & Sons, 1997.

*Härkki-Sirén, P. et al. "Finnish national register of laparoscopic hysterectomies: a review and complications of 1165 operations." *American Journal of Obstetrics and Gynecology* 176(1 Pt 1) (January 1997): 118–122.

*Härkki-Sirén, P. et al. "Urinary tract injuries after hysterectomy." *Obstetrics and Gynecology* 92(1) (July 1998): 113–118.

*Hill, D.A. "Laparoscopy," obgyn.net, www.obgyn.com.

*Hutchins, F.L. "Abdominal myomectomy as a treatment for symptomatic uterine fibroids." *Obstetrics and Gynecology Clinics of North America* 22 (1995): 781–789.

*Hysteroscopes and Gynecological Laparoscopes, Submission Guidance for a 510(k)." March 7, 1996. Prepared by: Obstetrics-Gynecology Devices Branch, Office of Device Evaluation, Center for Devices and Radiological Health (FDA).

*Landi, S. et al. "Laparoscopic myomectomy: technique, complications, and ultrasound scan evaluations." *Journal of the American Association of Gynecological Laparoscopists* 8(2) (May 2001): 231–240.

*Lipman, J.C. "Uterine Artery Embolization for the Treatment of Symptomatic Uterine Fibroids: A Review." *Applied Radiology* 29(7) (2000): 15–20.

*Mayfield, E. "Choosing a Treatment for Uterine Fibroids." *FDA Consumer Magazine* (October 15, 1997).

*Nathorst-Boos, J. et al. "Consumer's attitude to hysterectomy. The experience of 678 women." *Acta Obstetricia et Gynecologica Scandinavica* 71(3) (April 1992): 230–234.

*Nezhat, C. "The 'cons' of laparoscopic myomectomy in women who may reproduce in the future." *International Journal of Fertility and Menopausal Studies* 41(3) (May–June 1996): 280–283.

*Nezhat, F.R. et al. "Recurrence rate after myomectomy." *Journal of the American Association of Gynecologic Laparoscopists* 15 (1998): 237–240.

*Slupik, R.I. *American Medical Association Complete Guide to Women's Health*. New York: Random House, 1996.

*Smith, S.J. "Uterine Fibroid Embolization." *American Family Physician* *www.aafp.org/afp/20000615/3601.html*. 6/15/2000.

*Sudik, R. et al. "Fertility and pregnancy outcome after myomectomy in sterility patients." *European Journal of Obstetrics, Gynecology, and Reproductive Biology* 65(2) (April 1996): 209–214.

*"Uterine Leiomyomata." *ACOG Educational Bulletin* Number 192 (May 1994).

*Vercellini, P. et al. "Abdominal myomectomy for infertility: a comprehensive review." *Human Reproduction* 13(4) (April 1998): 873–879.

*Verkauf, B.S. "Myomectomy for fertility enhancement and preservation." *Fertility and Sterility* 58(1) (July 1992): 1–15.

*"VersaPoint System for Fibroid Removal Cleared by FDA." *www.plsgroup.com*. 11/4/96.

Month 11

*Agency for Healthcare Research and Quality. *Management of Uterine Fibroids*. Summary, Evidence Report/Technology Assessment: Number 34. AHRQ Publication No. 01-E051 (January 2001).

*Angier, N. *Woman*. Boston: Houghton Mifflin, 1999.

*Balfour, R.P. "Laparoscopic assisted vaginal hysterectomy—190 cases: complications and training." *Journal of Obstetrics and Gynecology* vol. 19, no. 2 (March 1999): 164–166.

*Broder, M.S. et al. "Uterine Artery Embolization: A Systematic Review of the Literature and Proposal for Research." The Rand Corp.: 5, 6, 21.

*Browder, S.E. "Hysterectomy and Your Heart." *Woman's Day* (in association with the American Heart Association) (April 24, 2001): 52–58.

*Carlson, K.J. et al. "The Maine Women's Health Study I: Outcomes of hysterectomy." *Obstetrics and Gynecology* 83(4): 556–572.

*Chopelas, A. "Fibroid Study and Research Program: Causes, Symptoms, Relief and Possible Solutions." 1997, originally published on Intradesign.com.

*Cellini, E.B. *Autobiography*. The Harvard Classics, 1909–14, *www.bartleby.com/31/1028.html#note1.28.1*.

*"Common Uterine Conditions," U.S. Dept. of Health and Human Services, AHCPR Publication No.98-0003, December 1997: 2.

*Cornforth, T. "Hysterectomy—Is it really necessary?" *womenshealth.guide@miningco.com*. 11/23/97.

*Davies, A. et al. "Indications and alternatives to hysterectomy." *Baillieres Clinical Obstetrics and Gynaecology* 11(1) (March 1997): 61–75.

*Falkeborn, M. et al. *Journal of Clinical Epidemiology* 53(8) (August 2000): 832–837.

*"Fertility, Family Planning, and Women's Health: New Data From the 1995 National Survey of Family Growth," May 1997 Vital and Health Statistics, Centers for Disease Control and Prevention/National Center for Health Statistics, U.S. Department of Health and Human Services, Series 23 No. 19, Table 52:62.

*The Fibroid Embolization Center, *www.uhmc.com/fibroid.htm*.

*Frieden, J. "Hysterectomy Patients May Face Incontinence Later." WebMD Medical News, *http://my.webmd.com/condition_center_content/whp/article/1728.60390*. 8/15/00.

*Galen, D.J. et al. "Outpatient Laparoscopic Hysterectomy: A Review of 50 Patients." *Journal of the American Association of Gynecologic Laparoscopists* (May 1994).

*Goldfarb, H.A. et al. *The No-Hysterectomy Option: Your Body—Your Choice*. New York: John Wiley & Sons, 1997.

*Härkki-Sirén, P. "Laparoscopic Hysterectomy." *http://ethesis.helsinki.fi/julkaisut/laa/naist/vk/harkki-siren/discussion.html*.

*Härkki-Sirén, P. "Review of the Literature, History of Hysterectomy." *http://ethesis.helsinki.fi/julkaisut/laa/naist/vk/harkki-siren/review.html*.

*Helstrom, L. et al. "Sexuality after hysterectomy: a factor analysis of women's sexual lives before and after subtotal hysterectomy." *Obstetrics and Gynecology* 81(3) (March 1993): 357–362.

*Hensel, B. "Hysterectomy Should Be Last Resort." *www.nbc4.tv*.

*"Hysterectomy." *www.plainsense.com/Health/Women's/hystrctm.htm*.

*"Hysterectomy: Know Your Options." National Women's Health Report, vol. 16, no. 3 (April 1994).

*Kritz-Silverstein, D. et al. "Hysterectomy, oophorectomy, and heart disease risk factors in older women." *American Journal of Public Health* 87(4) (April 1997): 676–680.

*Lepine, L.A. et al. *Hysterectomy Surveillance—United States, 1980–1993*. Division of Reproductive Health, National Center for Chronic Disease Prevention and Health Promotion, Centers for Disease Control and Prevention vol. 46, no. SS-4; 1–15 (August 8, 1997).

*Lipman, J.C. "Uterine Artery Embolization for the Treatment of Symptomatic Uterine Fibroids: A Review." *Applied Radiology* 29(7) (2000): 15–20.

*Luoto, R. et al. "Cardiovascular morbidity in relation to ovarian function after hysterectomy." *Obstetrics and Gynecology* 85(4) (April 1995): 515–522.

*Magos, A. et al. "Vaginal hysterectomy for the large uterus." *British Journal of Obstetrics and Gynaecology* 103(3) (March 1996): 246–251.

*Mayfield, E. "Choosing a Treatment for Uterine Fibroids." *FDA Consumer Magazine* (October 15, 1997).

*Meltomaa, S.S. et al. "One-year cohort of abdominal, vaginal, and laparoscopic hysterectomies: complications and subjective outcomes." *Journal of the American College of Surgeons* 189(4) (October 1999): 389–396.

*Munro, M.G. "Supracervical hysterectomy: . . . a time for reappraisal." *Obstetrics and Gynecology* 89(1) (January 1997): 133–139.

*Nathorst-Boos, J. et al. "Psychological reactions and sexual life after hysterectomy with and without oophorectomy." *Gynecologic and Obstetric Investigation* 34(2) (1992): 97–101.

*Northrup, C. *Women's Bodies, Women's Wisdom*. New York: Bantam Books, 1994.

*Parikh, J.P. et al. "Outcome Following Subtotal Hysterectomy." *Journal of Obstetrics and Gynecology* vol. 20, no. 1 (January 2000): 70–73.

*Podolsky, D. "Saved From the Knife." *U.S. News and World Report* 109(20) (1990): 76–77.

*Polet, R. et al. "Laparoscopically assisted vaginal hysterectomy (LAVH)—an alternative to total abdominal hysterectomy." *South Africa Medical Journal* 86(9 Suppl) (September 1996): 1190–1194.

*Raboch, J. et al. "Sex life following hysterectomy," *Geburtshilfe und Frauenheilkunde* 45(1) (January 1985): 48–50.

*Rako, S. "Testosterone supplemental therapy after hysterectomy with or without concomitant oophorectomy: estrogen alone is not enough." *Journal of Women's Health and Gender Based Medicine* 9(8) (October 2000): 917–923 Ê.

*Rhodes, J.C. et al. "Hysterectomy and Sexual Functioning." *JAMA* vol. 282, no. 20 (November 24, 1999): 1934–1941.

*Sakai, K. et al. "Female sexual response after hysterectomy." *Nippon Sanka Fujinka Gakkai Zasshi* 35(6) (June 1983): 757–763.

*Shoupe, D. "Hysterectomy or an Alternative?" *Hospital Practice* http://www.hosppract.com/issues/2000/09/shoupe.htm.

*Society for Women's Health Research. "Survey Shows Two-Thirds of Women are Unaware of Alternatives to Hysterectomy for Treating Excessive Menstrual Bleeding." www.womens-health.org. 11/28/00.

*Stoney, C.M. et al. "A natural experiment on the effects of ovarian hormones on cardiovascular risk factors and stress reactivity: bilateral salpingo oophorectomy versus hysterectomy only." *Health Psychology* 16(4) (July 1997): 349–358.

*"The Uterus: Still a Mystery." Wellness Web, www.wellweb.com.

*Toufexis, A. "Preserving Fertility While Treating Cervical Cancer," *The New York Times*, 31 July 2001).

*Vedantham, S. et al. "Uterine Artery Embolization for Fibroids: Considerations in Patient Selection and Clinical Follow-up." Medscape Women's Health 4(5), www.medscape.com/Medscape/WomensHealth/journal/1999/v04.n05. 1999.

*Vietz, P.F. "Hysterectomy—Historical perspective," www.qis.net. 9/97.

*Weaver, F. et al. "Hysterectomy in Veterans Affairs Medical Centers." *Obstetrics and Gynecology* 97(6) (June 2001): 880–884.

*West, S. *The Hysterectomy Hoax*. New York: Main Street Books, Doubleday, 1994.

*Weston, L.C. "Hysterectomy Can Have an Impact on Sexuality." ONHEALTH, www.onhealth.com/ch1/Columnist/Item,15017.asp. 9/17/98.

Month 12

*Agency for Healthcare Research and Quality. *Management of Uterine Fibroids*. Summary, Evidence Report/Technology Assessment: Number 34. AHRQ Publication No. 01-E051 (January 2001).

*Firstman, R. "Heal Thyself." *Time/ON* Magazine (March 5, 2001): 3.

*Hilts, P.J. "Web Sites Inconsistent on Health, Study Finds," *The New York Times*, 23 May 2001.

*Landro, L. "Online Health Groups Step Up Attempts to Enforce Standards," *The Wall Street Journal*, 20 July 2001, p. B1.

Acknowledgments

FIRST OF all, thanks and grateful acknowledgment to my editor, Matthew Lore, for inviting me to be part of his *The First Year*™ series. I'm proud to be part of Matthew's vision of providing resources for the newly diagnosed. I would also like to thank Sue McCloskey, Ghadah Alrawi, David Reidy, and Linda Kosarin at the Avalon Publishing Group, Pauline Neuwirth at Neuwirth & Associates for her text design, and Howard Grossman for his cover design.

Thanks also to my agent, Andrea Pedolsky, for her continuing encouragement; friendship, support, and guidance.

Special thanks to Katherine Kurs for her invaluable and hard-won tips on preparing for hospital stays, and to Dr. Nelson Stringer for providing the foreword.

And to my very own Support Team (and not just for fibroids) . . . among them, Rochelle Cohen, Don Cohen, Susan Sanders, Susan Carr, Sandi Borger, Ellen Fisher Turk, Andrew Koopman, John Hudson, Jacob Bender, Carey Earle, Cathleen Ritterreiser, Lia Bass, Debra Joyce, Howard Matz, Stephen Altman, Javier and Rebecca Rosenzwaig, Claudio and Robin Kolodzinski, Amber Wood, Mitchell Markson, Anno Mungen,

Robert Rosenlund, Joan Siegel, Ellen Lesser, Jeff Krauss, Laurie Baum, Milton Wainberg, Elizabeth Rubin, Sharon Linnea, David Leipziger, Bobbi Berenbaum, Larry Mark, Simone Franco, Eileen Weiss, Andrea Schwartz, Bob Brashear, Fern and Danny Flamberg, David and Lois Cohen, Matt and Marla Herman, Betty Herman, Lis and Tom Hogan, Mom and Dad, and very importantly, Zachary, Allison, Josh, Marlene, and Lilly, for being the firma in my terra.

In loving memory of Marshall T. Meyer, Grandma Siegel, and Uncle Sid, who always expected good things from me.

And finally, I'd like to thank you, for taking care of yourself, for joining the community of women who are knowledgeable about fibroids, and perhaps for sharing your new knowledge with someone else who will be grateful for your insights, comfort, and support.

With best wishes for health, happiness, and peace of mind,

Johanna

Index